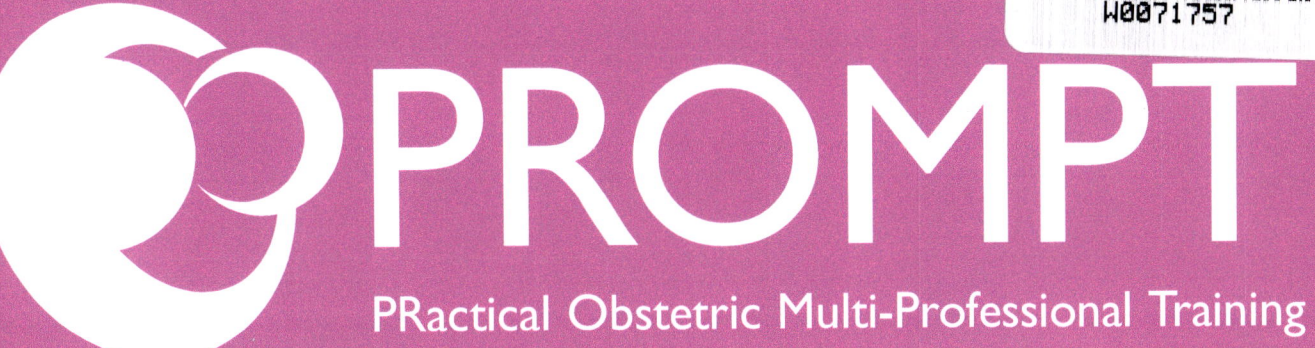

PROMPT

PRactical Obstetric Multi-Professional Training

Course Manual

North American edition

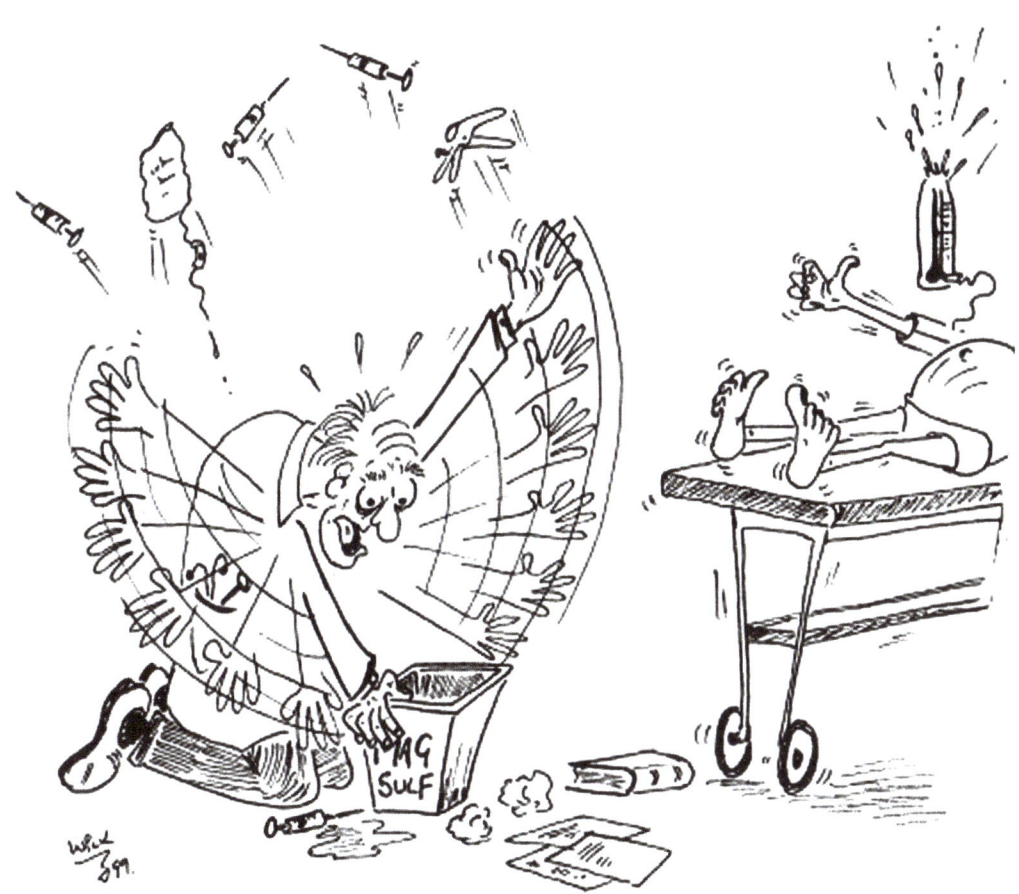

Edited by

Carl P. Weiner

PROMPT

PRactical Obstetric Multi-Professional Training

Practical locally based training for obstetric emergencies

Course Manual
North American edition

Edited by

Carl P. Weiner

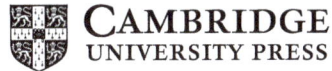

CAMBRIDGE UNIVERSITY PRESS

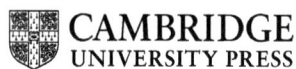

Shaftesbury Road, Cambridge CB2 8EA, United Kingdom

One Liberty Plaza, 20th Floor, New York, NY 10006, USA

477 Williamstown Road, Port Melbourne, VIC 3207, Australia

314–321, 3rd Floor, Plot 3, Splendor Forum, Jasola District Centre, New Delhi – 110025, India

103 Penang Road, #05–06/07, Visioncrest Commercial, Singapore 238467

Cambridge University Press is part of Cambridge University Press & Assessment, a department of the University of Cambridge.

We share the University's mission to contribute to society through the pursuit of education, learning and research at the highest international levels of excellence.

www.cambridge.org
Information on this title: www.cambridge.org/9781107549548

First published in the UK 2008; second UK edition published in 2013

North American edition published 2016

First published 2016

A catalogue record for this publication is available from the British Library

Library of Congress Cataloging-in-Publication data
Names: Weiner, Carl P., editor. | PROMPT Maternity Foundation, issuing body.
Title: PROMPT : PRactical Obstetric Multi-Professional Training : practical locally based training for obstetric emergencies course manual / North American edition edited by Carl P. Weiner.
Other titles: PRactical Obstetric Multi-Professional Training
Description: North American edition. | Cambridge, United Kingdom ; New York : Cambridge University Press, 2016. | First published in the UK 2008. | Includes bibliographical references and index.
Identifiers: LCCN 2015046462 | ISBN 9781107549548 (pbk. : alk. paper)
Subjects: | MESH: Obstetric Labor Complications | Pregnancy Complications | Obstetrics–education | Emergencies | Outlines | Problems and Exercises
Classification: LCC RG571 | NLM WQ 18.2 | DDC 618.2/025076–dc23 LC record available at http://lccn.loc.gov/2015046462

ISBN   978-1-107-54954-8   Paperback

....

Contents

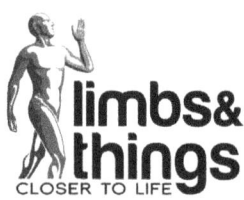
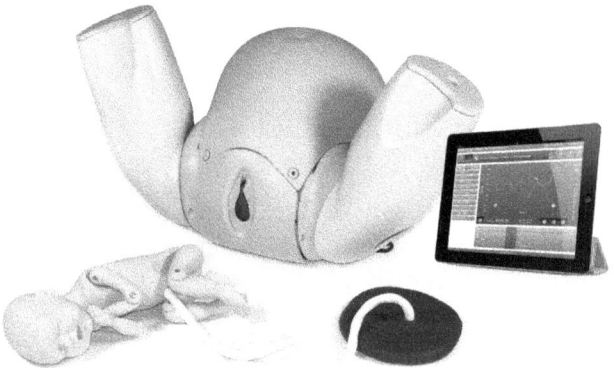
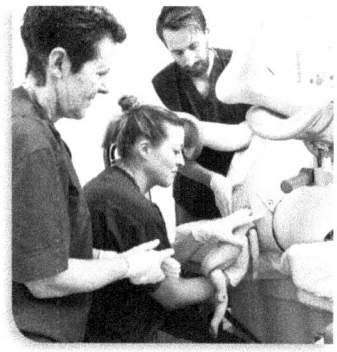
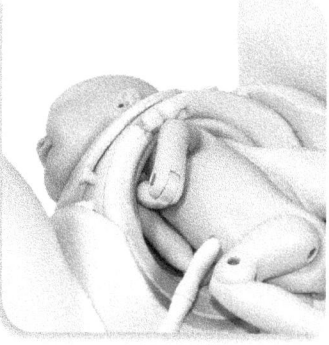
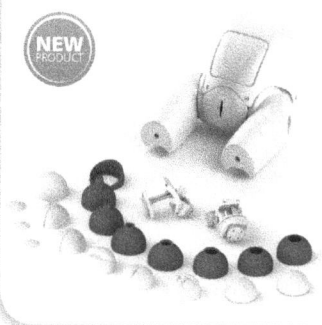

Contributors

Original contributors

Lt. Col. Tracy-Louise Appleyard — Consultant Obstetrician and Gynaecologist, Bristol/RAMC, UK

Mr. George Attilakos — Consultant Obstetrician, London, UK

Dr. Sonia Barnfield — Consultant Obstetrician, Bristol, UK

Ms. Christine Bartlett — Senior Midwife, Gloucester, UK

Dr. Joanna Crofts — Clinical Lecturer, University of Bristol, UK

Dr. Fiona Donald — Consultant Anaesthetist, Bristol, UK

Professor Timothy Draycott — Consultant Obstetrician, Bristol, UK

Dr. Sian Edwards — Research Registrar, Bristol, UK

Ms. Denise Ellis — Senior Midwife, Bristol, UK

Mr. Christopher Eskell — PROMPT Maternity Foundation, Executive Member

Mr. Robert Fox — Consultant Obstetrician, Taunton, UK

Mr. Simon Grant — Consultant Obstetrician, Bristol, UK

Dr. Judith Hyde — Consultant Obstetrician, Bristol, UK

Mr. Mark James — Consultant Obstetrician and Gynaecologist, Gloucester, UK

Ms. Sharon Jordan — Senior Midwife, Bristol, UK

Dr. Christina Laxton — Consultant Anaesthetist, Bristol, UK

Ms. Sharyn Mckenna — Maternity Risk Manager, Bristol, UK

Dr. Neil Muchatuta — Consultant Anaesthetist, Bristol, UK

Dr. Kate O'Brien — Specialty Registrar in Obstetrics & Gynaecology, Bristol, UK

Dr. David Odd — Consultant Neonatologist, Bristol, UK

Ms. Beverley Osborne	Senior Midwife, Bristol, UK
Ms. Helen Ping	Senior Midwife, Bristol, UK
Dr. Alison Pike	Consultant Neonatologist, Bristol, UK
Dr. Mark Scrutton	Consultant Anaesthetist, Bristol, UK
Ms. Debbie Senior	Practice Development Midwife, Bristol, UK
Dr. Dimitris Siassakos	Clinical Lecturer, University of Bristol, UK
Mr. Thabani Sibanda	Consultant Obstetrician, New Zealand
Dr. Rebecca Simms	Research Registrar, Bristol, UK
Ms. Angie Sledge	Senior Midwife, Bristol, UK
Dr. Nicky Weale	Consultant Anaesthetist, Bristol, UK
Ms. Heather Wilcox	Senior Midwife, Bristol, UK
Ms. Cathy Winter	PROMPT Maternity Foundation Midwife, UK
Dr. Anoushka Winton	Specialty Trainee in Anaesthesia
Ms. Stephanie Withers	Labour Ward Matron, Bristol, UK
Ms. Elaine Yard	Senior Midwife, Bristol, UK
Mr. Andy Yelland	Senior Midwife, Bristol, UK
Ms. Mandi Yelland	Senior Midwife, Bristol, UK

North American edition contributors

Dr. Andrew Malinow	Obstetric Anesthesiology, University of Maryland, USA
Dr. Prabhu Parimi	Neonatology, University of Kansas, USA
Ms. Michelle Schultz	Obstetric Unit Coordinator, University of Kansas, USA
Ms. Elise Van Daalen	Nurse Practitioner, University of Kansas, USA

Acknowledgments

PROMPT North America is a not-for-profit corporation registered in Delaware. The PROMPT Maternity Foundation (PMF) is a registered charity in England and Wales (Charity No. 1140557). The aim of the charity is to improve awareness and facilitate the distribution of effective obstetric emergencies training as widely as possible, to areas of the world requesting access to an economical and sustainable training model. This is a significant project aimed at reducing maternal and perinatal morbidity and mortality.

The original PROMPT Course Manual was developed and produced with the support of:

- Staff of North Bristol NHS Trust, UK
- The South West Obstetric Network, UK
- All researchers, facilitators and participants of the SaFE Study (Department of Health, UK)
- Limbs and Things, Bristol, UK
- Laerdal Medical, Norway
- Ferring Pharmaceuticals, UK

The final production of the PROMPT Course in a Box would not have been possible without the invaluable help and support of:

- The Louise Stratton Memorial Fund
- Colstons Girls School, Bristol, UK
- Mrs. Lewis, Bristol, UK
- Meg Winter, Bristol, UK

PROMPT training is endorsed by:

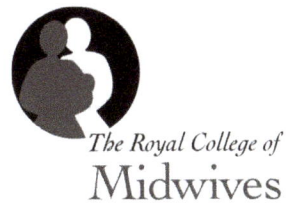

Royal College of
Obstetricians and Gynaecologists

Bringing to life the best in women's health care

Obstetric
Anaesthetists'
Association

List of abbreviations and terms

ABC	airway, breathing, circulation
ABCDE	airway, breathing, circulation, displacement, exposure
ACLS	advanced cardiac life support
AED	automated external defibrillator
ALT	alanine aminotransferase
APH	antepartum hemorrhage
aPTT	activated partial thromboplastin time
AST	aspartate aminotransferase
BP	blood pressure
bpm	beats/minute
BUN	blood urea nitrogen
Ca^{2+}	calcium
CAB	circulation, airway, breathing
CBC	complete blood count
CESDI	Confidential Enquiry into Stillbirths and Deaths in Infancy
CMACE	Centre for Maternal and Child Enquiries
CNST	Clinical Negligence Scheme for Trusts
CO_2	carbon dioxide
CPR	cardiopulmonary resuscitation
CT	computed tomography
CVA	cerebrovascular accident
DIC	disseminated intravascular coagulation
ECV	external cephalic version
EFM	electronic fetal heart rate monitoring
EKG	electrocardiogram

FFP .... fresh frozen plasma

FHR .... fetal heart rate

HELLP syndrome .... hemolysis, elevated liver enzymes, and low platelets

HIE .... hypoxic ischemic encephalopathy

HIV .... human immunodeficiency virus

ICU .... intensive care unit

IM .... intramuscular

IV .... intravenous

K^+ .... potassium

LFT .... liver function test

LMA .... laryngeal mask airway

MBRRACE-UK .... Mothers and Babies: Reducing Risk through Audits and Confidential Enquiries in the UK

MOEWS .... modified obstetric early warning score

MRI .... magnetic resonance imaging

Na^+ .... sodium

NICE .... National Institute for Health and Care Excellence

NICHD .... National Institute of Child Health and Human Development

NPSA .... National Patient Safety Agency

$PaCO_2$ .... arterial partial pressure of carbon dioxide

PaO_2 .... arterial partial pressure of oxygen

PEA .... pulseless electrical activity

PPH .... postpartum hemorrhage

PROMPT .... Practical Obstetric Multi-professional Training

SBAR .... situation, background, assessment, and recommendation/response

VBAC .... vaginal birth after cesarean

VF .... ventricular fibrillation

VT .... ventricular tachycardia

WBC .... white blood cell count

WOMAN trial .... World Maternal Antifibrinolytic trial

Foreword to the first edition

The world's attention is on the Millennium Development Goals (MDGs). MDG 4 aims to reduce child mortality, of which 50% are newborns, and MDG 5 aims to reduce maternal mortality. Pregnancy, labor, and birth are in the most part safe, but some births are not as safe as they could or should be.

The research of the PROMPT Maternity Foundation and its members has confirmed that leadership and multi-professional teamworking, together with the appropriate knowledge and clinical skills, are essential to provide the best care for the mother and the fetus/newborn and thus to achieve MDGs 4 and 5. PROMPT provides just such training and has been associated with improvements in perinatal outcomes.

The PROMPT training package consists of a "Course in a Box," which includes a Course Manual, a Trainer's Manual, and a CD-ROM of lectures and videos. It provides course materials to enable local staff to run "in-house" multi-professional obstetric emergencies courses in their own maternity units or other local settings.

The training package is written by a team of expert researchers who have many years of experience of conducting PROMPT training both locally and around the world. The evaluation of the effectiveness of the training with regard to its associated improvements in clinical outcomes is a priority of the PROMPT team. This scientific evidence is the hallmark of PROMPT.

Improving safety and quality by better knowledge, skills, teamwork, and leadership is our responsibility. I am sure those who attend the PROMPT training program and use the PROMPT materials will be able to deliver safe, high-quality care.

Sir Sabaratnam Arulkumaran,
President, International Federation of
Gynecology and Obstetrics

September 2015

Module 1
Teamworking (human factors)

Key learning objectives

- Understand the importance of good teamworking.
- Understand that effective communication is vital in emergency situations.
- Understand the importance of stating the problem early at the outset of the communication.
- Appreciate the different roles and responsibilities of members comprising a multi-professional team.
- Understand the importance of shared decision making within the team.
- Recognize the value of situational awareness – the ability to "stand back and take a broader view" in an emergency.

Introduction

Severe maternal morbidity in North America continues to occur and, in fact, has increased in the United States since the late 1990s. Obstetric emergencies are unpredictable and sudden. Successful management requires a rapid and coordinated response by an often ad hoc multi-professional team. The need to provide training for clinicians in team coordination and communication has been repeatedly identified as a safety priority.

Although maternal deaths are the traditional indicator of maternal health outcomes, they are but the "tip of the iceberg." For every death, there are many women who have significant complications of pregnancy, labor, and delivery. Moreover, the most severe complications, such as acute renal failure, cardiac events, thromboembolism, and hemorrhage have increased dramatically in recent years.[1] Compared to prior years, the US pregnancy-related mortality ratio increased 2006 to 2010 as did the contribution of cardiovascular conditions and infection. More than 3,300 women died during that five-year period in association with pregnancy, placing the United States 60th in the world ranking for maternal deaths. The increasing contribution of chronic diseases to pregnancy-related mortality suggests a change in risk profile of the pregnant population.[2]

Some of the most granular information on adverse obstetric outcomes comes from other industrialized countries where organized review programs have operated for decades. Arguably the most comprehensive reviews are conducted in Great Britain. The most recent Centre for Maternal and Child Enquiries (CMACE) review noted 70% of direct maternal deaths were potentially preventable with better care;[3] a lack of multi-professional team working and communication failures were once again identified as contributory factors.[4,5] Prior Confidential Enquiries into Maternal Deaths identified poor communication and poor teamworking as major contributors to fetal and neonatal mortality.[6,7] And, in December 2014, MBRRACE concluded that in 52% of deaths, improvements in care may have made a difference. They make specific reference to failures in communication and teamwork.[8] Based on these and other reviews, numerous professional organizations and government panels have recommended obstetric emergencies training include teamworking.

Though much of the available literature is derived from UK studies, there is no reason to think that North America is any different. The 2004 Joint Commission Sentinel Alert Issue #30 reported on the root cause analysis of 71 sentinel events (61 deaths, 10 with severe morbidities). They identified problems with communication in 72% of cases, the safety culture in 55%, staff competency in 47%, and orientation and training in 40%.[9] They recommended all obstetrical healthcare organizations conduct:

- team training in perinatal areas to teach staff to work together and communicate more effectively
- clinical drills to help staff prepare for high-risk events
- debriefings to evaluate team performance.

In the UK, the Clinical Negligence Scheme for Trusts (CNST) Maternity Clinical Risk Management Standards (national negligence insurance) mandated there be a systematic process in maternity units ensuring multi-professional drill training for all relevant obstetric staff.[10]

Definitions

Teamwork is the combined, effective action of a group working towards a common goal. It requires that individuals with differing roles communicate effectively and work together in a coordinated fashion to achieve a successful outcome.

Teamwork training

Conventional healthcare training has typically focused on specific, technically skilled tasks. Yet, with the increasingly multi-professional nature of healthcare, a continued focus on individual knowledge, technical skills, and attitude may be inadequate.[11] Multi-professional team training for obstetric emergencies is associated with improved performance,[12] improved safety attitudes,[13] and improved perinatal outcomes.[14,15,16]

Teamwork training recognizes that people make fewer errors when they work in effective teams. Each member of the team better understands their responsibilities when processes are planned and standardized, with team members "looking out" for one another and correcting errors before they cause an accident.[17] This cannot occur when every team member has "their own way" of proceeding no matter how sound it may be.

There is also evidence that, even when training is conducted in multi-professional teams, some teams possess characteristics that make them more efficient than others, and they are better able to achieve good outcomes by performing key actions in a timely manner. These characteristics are not explained by differences in knowledge or skill,[8] emphasizing the need to include other aspects of teamworking to achieve optimal training outcomes.

Improvements in outcomes

As already mentioned, current evidence supports training for obstetric emergencies in multi-professional teams, the strongest evidence being the improved obstetric and perinatal outcomes after clinical training with integrated teamwork training.[18] However, not all training is equal, and some training programs have actually increased rates of poor perinatal outcomes rather than improving them.[19] Further, teamwork training conducted remotely from the daily practice site has not proven effective in obstetrics.[20,21]

The key features of training programs associated with improvements in perinatal outcome are:[14,17]

- training is conducted in-house
- 100% of healthcare staff that work in an obstetric unit train regularly
- all staff train together in teams consisting of the same professionals who normally work together and incorporate teamwork principles into clinical training scenarios
- system changes are introduced, reflecting feedback provided by staff after participating in the training.

In-house training appears the most efficient and cost-effective means of training all staff in an institution. In-house training also allows the team to identify unique local issues that can be used as a driver for system change.[10,14,22] Moreover, there is evidence that local training is the most effective way of improving outcomes.[23]

Finally, it appears the most efficient obstetric teams recognize and state verbally the emergency earlier, and have incorporated this critical task using closed-loop communication (task clearly and loudly delegated, accepted, executed, and completion acknowledged). For example, such teams administer magnesium sulfate within 10 minutes after an eclamptic seizure, have significantly fewer exits from the labor room, and use structured communication.[24] It is vital that such communication skills are integrated into clinical training.

Communication

Communication is the transfer of information and the sharing of meaning. Often, the purpose of communication is to clarify or acknowledge the receipt of the information. Since communication is frequently impaired under stress, it is important to learn techniques that increase awareness and help overcome this limitation.

There are five requirements for effective communication and efficient team performance:[25,26]

1. FORMULATED

Give a clear message. It should be succinct and not rambling. SBAR (Situation, Background, Assessment, and Recommendation/response) is a useful acronym for formulating messages and handing over information[20] and is used almost naturally by the most effective obstetric teams.[9,20] For example:

> Nurse Gulliver reports: "Jane Doe is septic (S). She is 33 weeks gestation with preterm, premature rupture of membranes

(PPROM) a week ago (B). She is in pain, hypotensive, and tachycardic. Her score is 3 on the modified obstetric early warning score (MOEWS) chart (A). I need help now. Please contact. . . . .(R)."

The use of MOEWS will be addressed in several subsequent modules. Figure 1.1 is an example of a maternal SBAR form that may be used when handing over information.

2. ADDRESSED TO SPECIFIC INDIVIDUALS (DELEGATED)

Use names of staff and make eye contact. Assign appropriate tasks to an identified person.

"Liz and Susan (labor nurses), please get Mrs. Jones into the McRoberts' position."

"Diane (labor nursing assistant), please record the times and actions as they are called out. Thanks."

3. DELIVERED

Messages are sent clearly, concisely, and calmly. When the emergency team arrives in your room, say:

"Susan Smith is having a postpartum hemorrhage. She has lost about a liter of blood. Her placenta delivered spontaneously and appeared complete. There was no episiotomy and her perineum is intact. She has a liter of normal saline with 40 units of oxytocin running wide open but her uterus still feels soft."

rather than:

"Oh wow, Susan has just had a really big baby. She has oxytocin running but she is bleeding, really bleeding. Can someone please help me?"

4. ACKNOWLEDGED

Adequate volume used and repeated back:

"Do you want to give methergine intramuscularly now?"

SBAR report to clinician about a clinical obstetric situation

S

Situation

I am calling about (woman's name): _____ Ward: _____ Hosp No: _____

The problem I am calling about is: _____

I have just made an assessment:

The vital signs are: Blood pressure ____ / ____ Pulse _____ Respirations_____ SPO$_2$ _____ % Temperature_____°C

I am concerned about:

Blood pressure because it is:
    systolic over 160
    diastolic over 100
    systolic less than 90
Pulse because it is:
    over 120
    less than 40
Respirations because they are:
    less than 10
    over 30
    The woman is having oxygen at
    _____ 1/min
Maternal temperature because it is: _____°C

Maternal serum lactate because it is: _____ mmol/1

Urine output because it is:
    less than 100mls over the last 4 hours
    significantly proteinuric (+++)
Hemorrhage:
    Antepartum
    Postpartum
Fetal wellbeing:
    Pathological EFM
FSS Result: pH _____
    Time sample taken: _____ hrs

Modified Obstetric Early Warning Chart Score: [ ] [ ]

B

Background (tick relevant section)

The woman is:
    Primiparous   Multiparous   Grand multiparous
    Gestation: _____ wks   Singleton   Multiple
    Previous Cesarean section or uterine surgery

Fetal wellbeing
    Abdominal palpation:
    Fundal height: _____cms   Presentation:_____   FH rate:_____bpm
    EFM: Normal   Suspicious   Pathological

Antenatal
    A/N problem (details): _____

Labor
    Spontaneous onset   Induced
    IUGR   Pre eclampsia   Reduced fetal movements   Diabetes   APH
    Oxytocin

    Most recent vaginal examination: Time _____hrs
    Cervical dilatation: _____cms   Station of presenting part:_____   Position: _____
    Membranes intact   Meconium stained   Fresh red loss
    Third stage complete   Retained placenta

Postnatal
    Delivery date: _____   Delivery time:_____hrs
    Type of delivery: _____   Perineal trauma:_____
    Blood loss: _____mls   Oxytocin infusion
    Fundus: High   Atonic   Uterus tender   Abdominal/perineal wound oozing

Treatment given / in progress: _____

A

Assessment

    I think the problem is: _____

    I am not sure what the problem is but the woman is deteriorating and we need to do something

R

Recommendation

    Request:
    Please come to see the woman immediately
    I think delivering needs to be expedited
    I think the woman needs to be transferred to delivery suite
    I would like advice please

Reported to: _____   **Response:** _____

Person completing form (name): _____Date:_____ Time: _____

SBAR Clinical Obstetric reporting sheet. Please photocopy form and file original in woman's notes and copy with Risk Incident form

Figure 1.1 Example SBAR handover sheet

5. ACTED UPON

Meaning acknowledged and action performed:

"OK. Methergine given IM at 15:30."

The use of non-verbal communication, including making eye contact with the targeted individual, helps prevent ambiguity and promotes a shared knowledge of intention. Improper terminology, slang, inaudible communication, excess chatter, and incomplete reports should be avoided.

Leadership: roles and responsibilities

Team leadership involves providing structure, direction, and support for other team members. The team leader is typically the most senior obstetrician present,[22] but may be a midwife, labor nurse, or an anesthesiologist – whoever knows the team members' roles and responsibilities and has adequate experience to anticipate the possible end to an emergency.[22] If there is any ambiguity, it is essential a team leader be nominated, declared verbally, and accepted by the rest of the team as soon as possible.[22]

Team leaders vary in their level of expertise for any particular emergency and also in their readiness to lead. While being the team leader requires a certain level of competence, it is unlikely they possess all the abilities of every team member present. Therefore the team leader's principal role is to coordinate the activities of the specialists within the team by communicating clearly and simply, delegating tasks appropriately, and planning ahead.[22] In addition, a good team leader respects the expertise of each team member, is willing to listen, and is open to criticism and constructive feedback.[22]

Other members of the team should have their individual roles identified and agreed to as early as possible. The leader should allocate critical tasks to specific team members, including a designated person to talk to the patient and her family.[22,27] Team members should be mutually supportive, communicate clearly, and give regular updates. They should avoid becoming fixated on minutiae or running around aimlessly.[20]

Situational awareness: the bigger picture

Situational awareness is how we notice, understand, and think ahead in a fast-paced, constantly changing situation. It is that "gut instinct" or "sixth sense" that makes a nurse, midwife, obstetrician, or anesthesiologist an expert. A situationally aware person recognizes and understands important cues, anticipates problems, and shares them with the team so that shared decision-making and goals are achieved.

Three levels of situational awareness are suggested.[28]

1. Notice

Be aware of the patient's status, the team members' status, and the available resources; anticipate possible errors by noticing cues and sharing decision-making:

> "The head nurse and a young obstetrician on call are reviewing the labor board, the floor is full and two of the women are ill: one is undelivered with severe pre-eclampsia and low urine output, and the other has had a 1,000 ml postpartum hemorrhage and an examination under anesthesia is planned. It is essential that both the nursing and obstetric leads for the shift are aware of the serious problems that may result. Only then can they anticipate and plan how to manage the cases and also consider which team members may be required to assist with the problems."

There is no such thing as a practitioner with a "white" cloud or a "black" cloud. Rather, there are only practitioners who are situationally aware and plan proactively, and those that are situationally unaware, reactive, and enter an emergency two steps behind.

2. Understand

Share information with the team, consider what the cues and clues may mean, be aware of common mistakes, re-evaluate/stand back at regular intervals, and seek to engage other team members in decisions.

> "After reviewing each of the cases, the head nurse and the young obstetrician identify several complicated problems that need decisions and action. They discuss whether to call the anesthesiologist to assist with the management of these potentially complicated patients. Before they can make this decision, they both go to each room for a thorough review, requesting an update from each of the nurses providing care. They then ask the opinion of the on-call anesthesiologist to gain further information that may influence the actions to be taken."

3. Think ahead

Anticipate, plan, and prioritize:

> "Having sought additional information and the opinions of other team members, the head nurse and the obstetrician are now able to identify potential problems, prioritize the cases, and form an action plan. Their ability to do so is based not only upon the information provided by the other team members but also on their own knowledge and previous experience. In this instance, they agree their first action should be to call a more senior obstetrician for management advice."

Situational awareness allows individuals to be "ahead of the game." Experienced clinicians usually have good situational awareness; they often pick up subtle cues, understand their significance, and use them to anticipate and pre-empt problems even if they cannot express them to a third party.[22] A recent MBRRACE report concluded after reviewing maternal deaths from hemorrhage that the main human factor was a lack of situational awareness, particularly in recognizing the severity of the problem in a timely fashion.[29]

Recognizing cues for loss of situational awareness

In extreme situations, people may "freeze," when their capacity to reason is so severely impaired by the stress of the workload that they are no longer able to function interactively with the rest of the team.

Characteristic signs of "freeze" include:

- poor communication
- inability to plan ahead
- tunnel vision
- fixation on irrelevant issues (such as less than ideal equipment) or displacement activities (such as unnecessary disputes with colleagues).

Even the presumed leader or good team players can completely "freeze up."

Maintaining/regaining situational awareness

One way of maintaining situational awareness is to adopt the philosophy of the "non-participant" leader: try not to become engaged in the practical tasks that can be performed by others. This allows the leader to take a step back and maintain a broader view of the unfolding emergency. In practice, this approach may be difficult as the team leader is often the team member with the particular "hands on" skills required for the problem.

Avoid panic. The following strategies can be tried to regain control of a situation:

- take a "helicopter view": stand back to get the bigger picture[22]
- declare an emergency early: you will engage everyone's attention and boost the available human resources. Early declaration is associated with improved clinical team performance and efficiency,[20] and can also improve the patient's perception of her care[23]
- communicate clearly and simply, starting with the critical tasks for each emergency[23]
- plan ahead: for example, prepare for a perimortem cesarean section in cases of maternal collapse
- delegate the critical tasks appropriately.[20]

Teamworking under pressure

Pressure situations create a sense of urgency – everything must be done immediately, increasing the tendency to rush. Rushing tasks under pressure increases the potential for errors. A good team leader tries to manage the emergency at a steady but efficient pace.

What makes a good team member?

- Good communicator
- Good understanding and acceptance of own limitations
- Awareness of environment and limitations of others
- Assertive
- Non-confrontational but willing to challenge if necessary
- Receptive to the suggestions of all other team members
- Thinks clearly

Key points

- Good team working is important since poorly functioning teams are associated with patient harm.
- Efficient teams state the emergency earlier and use closed-loop communication.
- Teamwork training may improve clinical outcomes when incorporated into clinical training.
- Multi-professional training locally (and ideally on-site) for all staff is associated with improved teamwork, improved safety attitudes, and, most importantly, improved perinatal outcomes.

References

1. Grobman WA, Bailit JL, Rice MM, Wapner RJ, Reddy UM, Varner MW, et al. Eunice Kennedy Shriver National Institute of Child Health and Human Development (NICHD) Maternal-Fetal Medicine Units (MFMU) Network. Frequency of and factors associated with severe maternal morbidity. *Obstet Gynecol* 2014;123: 804–10.

2. Creanga AA, Berg CJ, Syverson C, Seed K, Bruce FC, Callaghan WM. Pregnancy-related mortality in the United States, 2006–2010. *Obstet Gynecol* 2015; 125: 5–12.

3. Centre for Maternal and Child Enquiries. Saving Mothers' Lives: reviewing maternal deaths to make motherhood safer: 2006–08. *BJOG* 2011;118 Suppl 1: 1–203.

4. Lewis G (ed.). The Confidential Enquiry into Maternal and Child Health (CEMACH). *Saving Mothers' Lives: Reviewing Maternal Deaths to Make Motherhood Safer 2003–2005. The Seventh Report on Confidential Enquiries into Maternal Deaths in the United Kingdom*. London: CEMACH; 2007.

5. Lewis G (ed.). The Confidential Enquiry into Maternal and Child Health (CEMACH). *Why Mothers Die 2000–2002. The Sixth Report on Confidential Enquiries into Maternal Deaths in the United Kingdom*. London: RCOG Press; 2004.

6. Maternal and Child Health Research Consortium. *Confidential Enquiry into Stillbirths and Deaths in Infancy: 5th Annual Report, 1 January–31 December 1996*. London: Maternal and Child Health Research Consortium; 1998.

7. Maternal and Child Health Research Consortium. *Confidential Enquiry into Stillbirths and Deaths in Infancy: 7th Annual Report, 1 January–31 December 1998*. London: Maternal and Child Health Research Consortium; 2000.

8. Knight M, Kenyon S, Brocklehurst P, Neilson J, Shakespeare J, Kurinczuk JJ (eds) on behalf of MBRRACE UK. *Saving Lives, Improving Mothers' Care: Lessons Learned to Inform Future Maternity Care from the UK and Ireland Confidential Enquiries into Maternal Deaths and Morbidity 2009–12*. Oxford: National Perinatal Epidemiology Unit, University of Oxford; 2014.

9. Sentinel event alert issue 30: July 21, 2004. Preventing infant death and injury during delivery. *Adv Neonatal Care* 2004; 4: 180–1.

10. NHS Litigation Authority. *Clinical Negligence Scheme for Trusts: Maternity Clinical Risk Management Standards*. London: NHSLA; 2011 [www.nhsla.com/RiskManagement].

11. Siassakos D, Draycott TJ, Crofts JF, Hunt LP, Winter C, Fox R. More to teamwork than knowledge, skill and attitude. *BJOG* 2010; 117: 1262–9.

12. Siassakos D, Fox R, Crofts JF, Hunt LP, Winter C, Draycott TJ. The management of a simulated emergency: better teamwork, better performance. *Resuscitation* 2011; 82: 203–6.

13. Siassakos D, Fox R, Hunt L, Farey J, Laxton C, Winter C, et al. Attitudes toward safety and teamwork in a maternity unit with embedded team training. *Am J Med Qual* 2011; 26: 132–7.

14. Draycott T, Sibanda T, Owen L, Akande V, Winter C, Reading S, et al. Does training in obstetric emergencies improve neonatal outcome? *BJOG* 2006; 113: 177–82.

15. Draycott TJ, Crofts JF, Ash JP, Wilson LV, Yard E, Sibanda T, et al. Improving neonatal outcome through practical shoulder dystocia training. *Obstet Gynecol* 2008; 112: 14–20.

16. Weiner CP, Collins L, Bentley S, Dong Y, Satterwhite CL. Multi-professional training for obstetric emergencies in a US hospital over a 7-year interval: an observational study. *J Perinatol* 2016; 36: 19–24.

17. Helmreich RL. On error management: lessons from aviation. *BMJ* 2000; 320: 781–5.

18. Siassakos D, Crofts JF, Winter C, Weiner CP, Draycott TJ. The active components of effective training in obstetric emergencies. *BJOG* 2009; 116: 1028–32.

19. MacKenzie IZ, Shah M, Lean K, Dutton S, Newdick H, Tucker DE. Management of shoulder dystocia: trends in incidence and maternal and neonatal morbidity. *Obstet Gynecol* 2007; 110: 1059–68.

20. Nielsen PE, Goldman MB, Mann S, Shapiro DE, Marcus RG, Pratt SD, et al. Effects of teamwork training on adverse outcomes and process of care in labor and delivery: a randomized controlled trial. *Obstet Gynecol* 2007; 109: 48–55.

21. Riley W, Davis S, Miller K, Hansen H, Sainfort F, Sweet R. Didactic and simulation nontechnical skills team training to improve perinatal patient outcomes in a community hospital. *Jt Comm J Qual Patient Saf* 2011; 37: 357–64.

22. Thompson S, Neal S, Clark V. Clinical risk management in obstetrics: eclampsia drills. *Qual Saf Health Care* 2004; 13: 127–9.

23. Siassakos D, Crofts J, Winter C, Draycott T, on behalf of the SaFE Study Group. Multi-professional "fire-drill" training in the labour ward. *TOG* 2009; 11: 55–60.

24. Siassakos D, Bristowe K, Draycott TJ, Angouri J, Hambly H, Winter C, et al. Clinical efficiency in a simulated emergency and relationship to team behaviours: a multisite cross-sectional study. *BJOG* 2011; 118: 596–607.

25. Siassakos D, Draycott T, Montague I, Harris M. Content analysis of team communication in an obstetric emergency scenario. *J Obstet Gynaecol* 2009; 29: 499–503.

26. Bristowe K, et al. *Leadership and Teamwork for Clinical Emergencies: Multisite Interprofessional Focus Group Analysis*. Bristol: University of Bristol and University of the West of England; 2011.

27. Siassakos D, Bristowe K, Hambly H, Angouri J, Crofts JF, Winter C, et al. Team communication with patient actors: findings from a multisite simulation study. *Simul Healthc* 2011; 6: 143–9.

28. Endsley MR. The role of situation awareness in naturalistic decision making. In Zsambok CE, Klein G (eds) *Naturalistic Decision Making*. New Jersey, USA: Lawrence Erlbaum Associates; 1997. pp. 269–83.

29. Paterson-Brown S, Bamber J, on behalf of the MBRRACE-UK haemorrhage chapter writing group. Prevention and treatment of haemorrhage. In Knight M, Kenyon S, Brocklehurst P, Neilson J, Shakespeare J, Kurinczuk JJ (eds) on behalf of MBRRACE-UK. *Saving Lives, Improving Mothers' Care: Lessons Learned to Inform Future Maternity Care from the UK and Ireland Confidential Enquiries into Maternal Deaths and Morbidity 2009–12*. Oxford: National Perinatal Epidemiology Unit, University of Oxford 2014: p. 55.

Module 2
Basic life support and maternal collapse

Key learning points

- Assessment and resuscitation of maternal collapse:
  - ☐ CAB (circulation, airway, breathing)
- Manual left-uterine displacement or 30-degree left tilt if on firm tilting surface (e.g., operating table) to reduce aortocaval compression.
- Calling for help: effective communication of problem to the responding team.
- Equipment: knowing where to find the emergency cart and defibrillator.
- Appropriate documentation.

Common difficulties observed in training drills

- Failure to recognize cardiac arrest in a deteriorating patient.
- Not starting basic life support.
- Forgetting to keep the woman supine with manual left-uterine displacement.
- Forgetting to keep woman on a firm surface (use a rescue board especially if on a labor bed)
- Not administering high-flow oxygen to the mother.

Introduction

Maternal collapse occurs in a multitude of circumstances, and in obstetrics it is almost always unexpected. The presentation may range from an isolated and temporary drop in blood pressure to cardiac arrest and death. It is imperative that all healthcare professionals can provide basic life support, regardless of the cause. The 2004 Joint Commission Sentinel Alert Issue #30, which reported the root cause analysis of 71 sentinel events (61 deaths, 10 with severe morbidities), stressed the need for training after they observed that staff competency was an issue in 47%, and orientation and training in 40%.[1] They recommended that all obstetrical healthcare organizations conduct:

■ team training in perinatal areas to teach staff to work together and communicate more effectively

■ clinical drills to help staff prepare for high-risk events.

Resuscitation skills were considered poor in an unacceptably high number of the maternal deaths reviewed in 2007,[2] resulting in a recommendation that all clinical staff train regularly to improve basic, intermediate, and advanced life support skills. The need was repeated in 2014 by MBRRACE.[3]

Basic life support algorithm

All healthcare professionals should be able to perform basic life support. An outline of the basic life support algorithm is provided in Figure 2.1, but it is not intended to be a complete guide. Further information is available from the American Heart Association.[4]

What do we mean by maternal collapse?

Maternal collapse is severe respiratory or circulatory distress that may lead to a sudden change in level of consciousness, or cardiac arrest, if untreated. Any of the observations in Box 2.1 should trigger an emergency call for help.

Box 2.1 Observations that trigger an emergency response	
Airway	Obstructed or noisy
Breathing	Respiratory rate less than 5 or more than 35 breaths/minute
Circulation	Pulse rate less than 40 or more than 140 beats/minute
	Systolic blood pressure less than 80 or more than 180 mmHg
Neurology	Sudden decrease in level of consciousness
	Unresponsive or responsive to painful stimuli only
	Seizures

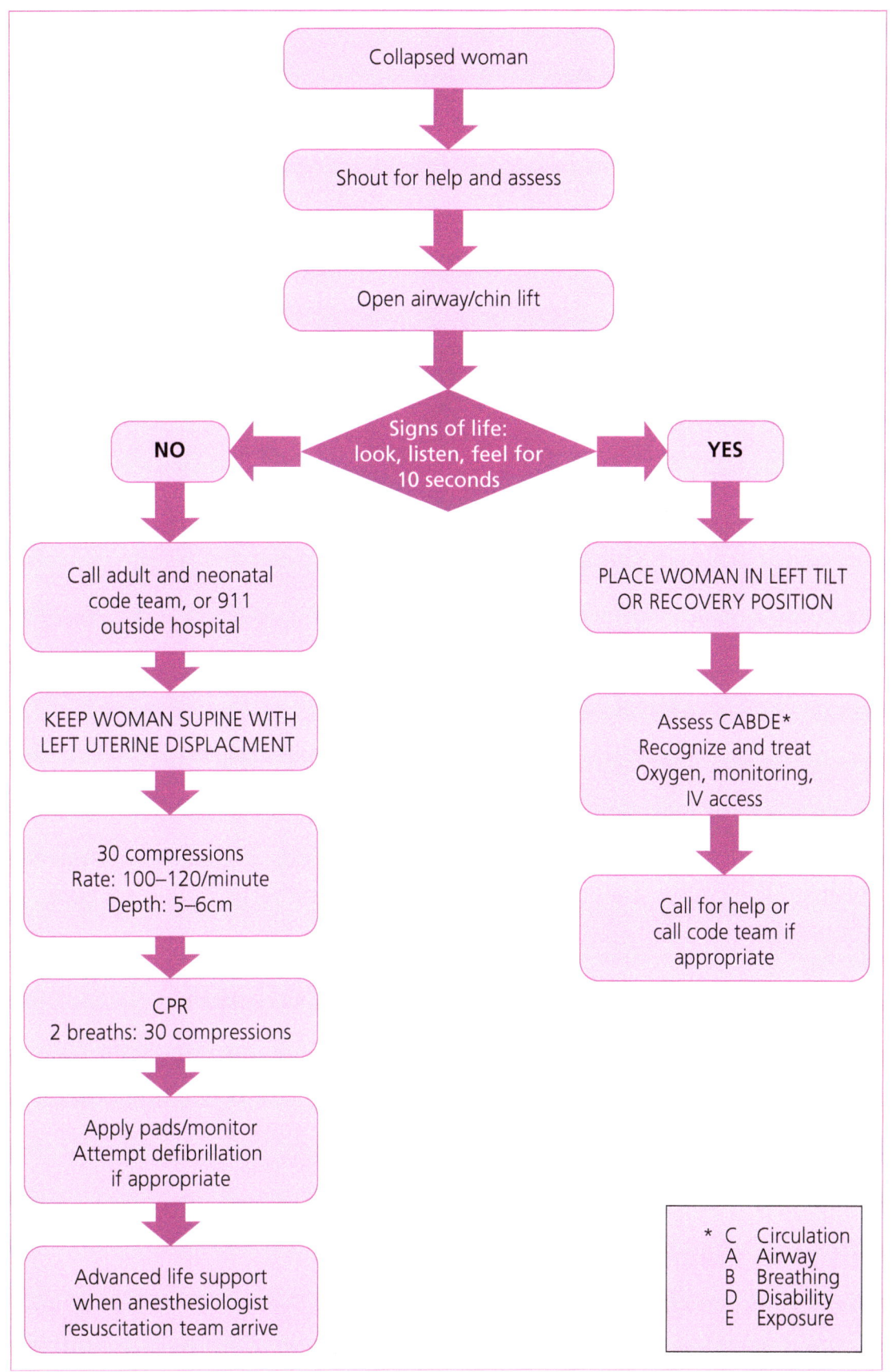

Figure 2.1 Basic life support algorithm

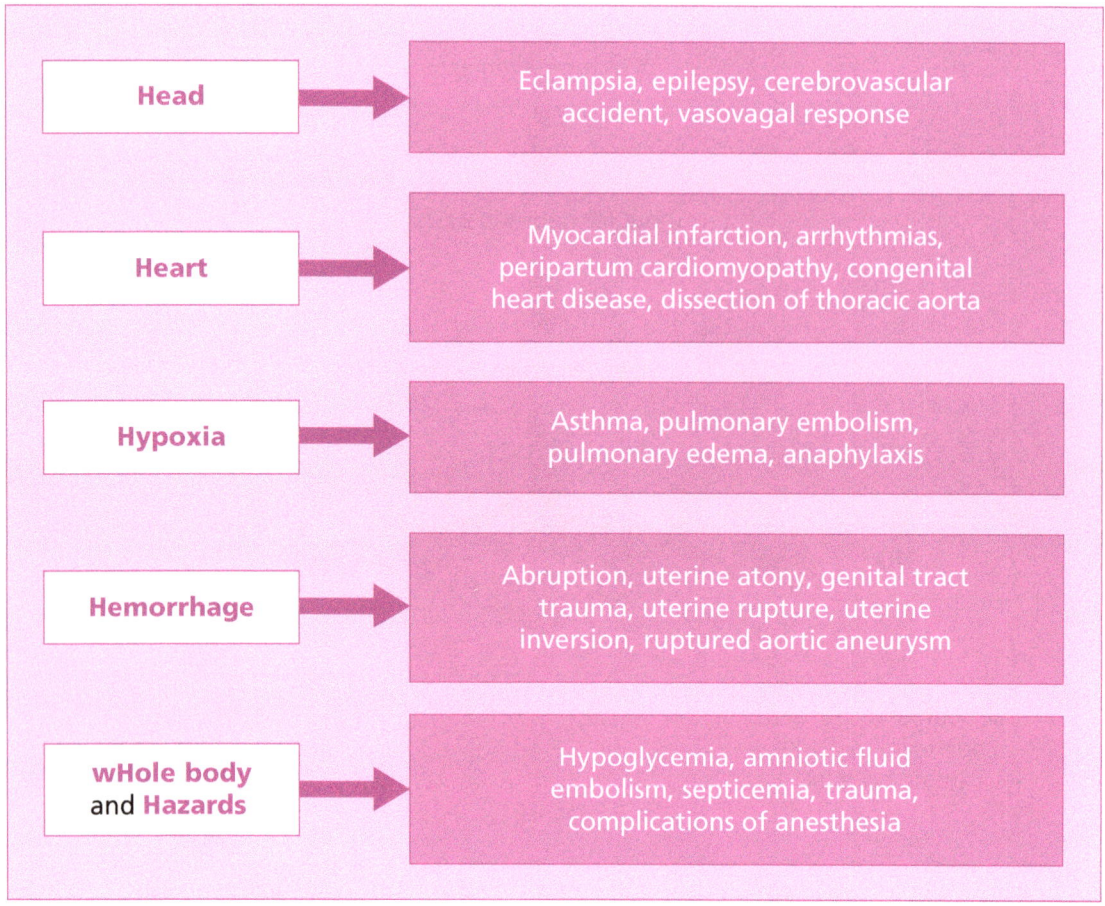

Figure 2.2 Possible causes of maternal collapse

Figure 2.2 illustrates a systematic way of classifying possible causes of maternal collapse. The causes are discussed in more detail in the following sections.

Management of maternal collapse

The key to the effective management of maternal collapse is a simple and structured approach to diagnosis and treatment. The underlying principles of the management of any critically ill patient are the same and are often described through the CAB approach (circulation, airway, breathing).

Initial management

- Assess the responsiveness of the woman by shaking her gently and asking if she is alright. If there is no response, immediately call for help using the emergency call button, dialing your hospital's code telephone number, or dialing 911 if you are outside hospital.

- Turn her on to her back and ask an assistant or passer by to manually displace the uterus leftward using one or two hands to reduce aortocaval obstruction (see Module 3: Figure 3.1). A 30-degree tilt can also be used if the woman is on a firm surface that can be tilted (e.g., an operating table). A firm resuscitation board should be inserted beneath the patient as soon as possible.

- Open the airway using head tilt and chin lift maneuvers.

- Assess breathing by looking for movement of the chest wall, listening for breath sounds, and feeling the exhaled air on your cheek (look, listen, feel) for up to 10 seconds. Agonal gasps (isolated or infrequent gasping in the absence of other breathing in an unconscious person) occur in the first minutes after sudden cardiac arrest; they are an indication to start cardio-pulmonary resuscitation (CPR) immediately and should not be confused with normal breathing.

- While assessing breathing, observe for other signs of life, such as color and movement.

- If there is no sign of life, call for help and commence basic life support without delay (Figure 2.1) until help arrives (to provide advanced life support) or the woman shows signs of life.

- If there are signs of life, place her in the recovery position and give high-flow oxygen via a reservoir mask. Obtain intravenous access, take blood samples (complete blood count, partial prothrombin and prothrombin clotting tests, urea and electrolytes, glucose, liver function tests, blood type, and hold) and initiate intravenous fluids. Monitor the electrocardiogram (EKG), and record respirations, pulse, blood pressure measurement, and transcutaneous oxygen saturation.

Primary obstetric survey

A primary obstetric-oriented survey is then performed, beginning at the head and working down to the feet. This process should generate a working diagnosis and allow initial treatment to begin. Box 2.2 shows the questions to be considered when performing the primary obstetric survey. It is important you seek support from the most experienced obstetrician and anesthesiologist available if not already present.

Decide on continuing treatment

The cause of the collapse and the treatment required may be evident after the primary survey; for example, eclampsia or hemorrhage. If the cause is not obvious, only a few key treatment decisions must be made.

Box 2.2 Primary obstetric survey	
Head	How responsive is the patient? Is she alert, does she respond to verbal commands, is she responsive to painful stimuli or unresponsive?
	Is she having a convulsion?
Heart	What is the capillary refill like?
	What is the pulse rate and rhythm?
	Is there a murmur?
Chest	Is there good bilateral air entry?
	What are the breath sounds like?
	Is the trachea midline?
Abdomen	Is there rebound and guarding?
	Is there tenderness (uterine or non-uterine)?
	Is the fetus alive?
	Is there a need for a laparotomy or delivery?
Vagina	Is there bleeding?
	What is the stage of labor?
	Is there an inverted uterus?

1. Is fluid resuscitation a priority or is it contraindicated? If in doubt, consider that fluid is usually beneficial: the exception is when the patient has, or is at great risk of, pulmonary edema, as may occur with severe pre-eclampsia or renal failure.

2. Is a laparotomy required for diagnosis or treatment? Is there evidence of an acute intra-abdominal event? Do you need to deliver the fetus to aid maternal resuscitation?

3. Is sepsis likely and are antibiotics a priority?

4. Is intensive care needed to provide airway, respiratory, or circulatory support?

Secondary obstetric survey

Further management will reflect the cause of the collapse. Once the patient has been stabilized, a secondary obstetric survey is performed (Box 2.3).

Box 2.3 Secondary obstetric survey	
ACTION	DETAIL
History	Review the history of the collapse and the patient's prior medical history
	Review the medical records and question her partner or relatives
Examine	Repeat the examination going from head to toe
Investigate	Obtain arterial blood gases, troponins, blood glucose, lactate, blood cultures, EKG, chest X-ray, ultrasound of the abdomen, and if relevant vaginal cultures
Monitor	Continue monitoring the EKG, respirations, pulse, blood pressure, and pulse oxymetry (if not already in use)
	Consider whether arterial and central venous pressure lines might aid monitoring
Pause and think further	Consider further investigations such as CT/MRI scans and echocardiography
	Ask relevant consultants for their opinions

Further key treatment decisions

Re-evaluate and continue to support the circulation, airway, and breathing. Do you need intensive care support? Continue to evaluate your working diagnosis periodically to ensure the pattern still fits and the selected treatment is working.

Specific causes of maternal collapse

Pulmonary thromboembolism

Pulmonary emboli are more common in pregnancy and the puerperium, owing to the procoagulant effect of pregnancy and blood flow stasis due to the combined vasodilation and mechanical obstruction by the uterus. Pulmonary emboli may be small and non-symptomatic, or large causing instant collapse and rapid death. In the United States, it is as common a cause of direct maternal death as hemorrhage, and the increased risk persists for up to a year after delivery.[5,6] Major risk factors include hyperemesis, multiple gestation, infection, and pre-eclampsia. Additional risk factors in the puerperium include obesity, cesarean delivery, and hemorrhage.[7]

Pulmonary emboli may present with shortness of breath, pleuritic chest pain, hemoptysis, or sudden collapse in a woman who may or may not have signs of a deep vein thrombosis. Clinical signs can include tachycardia, tachypnea, hypoxemia/hypoxia, and evidence of right heart strain on EKG (S1,Q3,T3) with a raised jugular venous pressure. Young women often present with only tachypnea with or without hypoxemia/hypoxia, so it is important to have a high index of suspicion. The initial assessment and treatment should be based on symptoms and signs plus analysis of arterial blood gases, EKG, and chest X-ray, with the diagnosis confirmed typically by computed tomography pulmonary angiography, or occasionally ventilation–perfusion scanning (VQ scan).

The initial treatment is supportive using oxygen by tight-fitting face mask, with ventilatory and cardiovascular support as necessary. Anticoagulation with heparin (subcutaneous low-molecular-weight heparin or intravenous unfractionated heparin) should be initiated quickly based on the clinical suspicion and continued until the diagnosis is confirmed or refuted.

Hemorrhagic shock

Hypovolemia, usually secondary to hemorrhage, is the most common cause of shock in obstetric patients. Signs of hypovolemia include:

- tachycardia and tachypnea
- cold, pale skin
- hypotension
- reduced urine output
- altered level of consciousness
- narrowed pulse pressure (<35 mmHg).

Prompt intravascular fluid replacement is essential. When there is significant hemorrhage, intra-arterial and central venous catheters (CVC) are often useful for maternal monitoring. A CVC provides access to the central circulation for vasoactive drugs as well as volume replacement. The etiology is typically obstetric in nature (e.g., uterine atony, abruption, ruptured uterus), but non-obstetric causes should also be considered.

While rare, aneurysm rupture may occur (such as aortic, renal, splenic, or iliac). Urgent laparotomy should be considered when there are signs of an acute abdomen in conjunction with hypovolemia.

Eclamptic seizures and coma

Eclamptic seizures and coma can resemble amniotic fluid embolus, but the presence of hypertension, proteinuria, and edema in the eclamptic woman differentiates the two. For more information about diagnosis and treatment, refer to Module 6.

Cerebrovascular accident

Cerebrovascular accidents (CVAs) may present with a wide range of neurological signs. CVAs can be embolic or hemorrhagic in origin. Hypertension, for example in severe pre-eclampsia, is a risk factor for CVA, and any pregnant woman with systolic blood pressure of 150 mmHg or greater requires antihypertensive treatment to reduce the risk of a CVA.[1] For more information on the management of acute hypertension during pregnancy, refer to Module 6. Migraine headaches can mimic CVAs. A CT or magnetic resonance imaging (MRI) scan can aid diagnosis and thus direct treatment. The recent MBRRACE report recommended neurological evaluation of all women with new onset headaches coupled with neck stiffness.[3]

Septic shock

Maternal sepsis was the second leading cause of death in the United States from 2006 through 2010 (second only to cardiovascular disease) and the number one cause of death in the UK from 2003 through 2005.[2,4] As many as 25% of the women who died, died from sepsis. It is crucially important that the symptoms and signs are recognized and acted upon directly. For more information about diagnosis and treatment, refer to Module 7.

Disseminated intravascular coagulation

Disseminated intravascular coagulation (DIC) may result from massive bleeding, severe infection, amniotic fluid embolism, or anaphylaxis. While pregnancy itself is a condition of chronic compensated DIC, any of the triggers may overwhelm the compensatory mechanisms resulting in a prolonged clotting time, low platelets, low fibrinogen, and hemorrhage. Spontaneous bleeding may occur from a needle puncture, intravenous cannula or epidural sites, as well as the woman's gums. Vaginal hemorrhage may also occur. It is important the blood bank along with the most experienced obstetrician and anesthesiologist available are involved early on with the management. Intensive care is vital if clinically symptomatic DIC is suspected. A blood sample for CBC, cross match, clotting tests, fibrinogen and D-dimers or fibrin degradation products should be sent. The cause of DIC should be investigated promptly and treated appropriately.

Hypo- or hyperglycemia

Women with diabetes may develop hypoglycemic coma. While rare, type 1 diabetes mellitus may develop during pregnancy. A blood glucose measurement should always be made in a collapsed or convulsing woman if the cause is not obvious, and her urine tested for ketones if diabetic ketoacidosis is suspected. Acute fatty liver may also present with maternal hypoglycemia. Administer 50 ml of 25% glucose solution intravenously if the blood glucose is found to be below 55 mg/dl (3 mmol/l) in a comatose woman.

Acute heart failure

Cardiac disease is the most common cause of direct and indirect maternal death in the United States.[4] A known history of cardiac disease, chest pain with EKG changes, or a new cardiac murmur may help to establish the diagnosis. If chest pain is a presenting feature, troponin levels should be obtained 6 hours after the onset of pain. Give 300 mg of aspirin orally if cardiac ischemia is suspected unless otherwise contraindicated. Arrange for a stat medical consultation and an echocardiogram if either cardiac failure be suspected or a new murmur is auscultated.

Pulmonary aspiration of gastric contents

Pregnancy increases the risk of pulmonary aspiration of stomach contents secondary to both progesterone-induced smooth muscle relaxation and delayed stomach emptying (a problem enhanced by labor) as well as mechanical effects on the esophageal sphincter. Aspiration is most likely to occur in the unconscious obstetric patient (for example, during an eclamptic convulsion or during induction/awakening from general anesthesia – delayed even in the post-anesthesia care unit) owing to the loss or suppression of the gag reflex. Aspiration may present with coughing, cyanosis, tachypnea, tachycardia, hypotension, or pulmonary edema.

Anaphylactic or toxic reaction to drugs or allergens

Anaphylactic or toxic reaction to drugs or allergens may present as convulsions or collapse. The close timing of administration of the drug or allergen (such as latex) in relation to the collapse may be the only clue for an anaphylactic or toxic reaction.

Severe anaphylaxis should be treated with:

- Oxygen 100% via mask with reservoir bag
- Epinephrine 500 mcg (0.5 ml of 1:1,000) IM (into side of thigh), repeated every 5 minutes if necessary
- Or, if an anesthesiologist is present, bolus doses of epinephrine (IV 50–100 mcg) up to 1 mg of a commercially prepared or diluted-at-bedside preparation (1 mg in 10 ml normal sterile saline to a concentration of 100 micrograms/ml or 1 in 10,000), and then
- Prepare other adjuvant drugs: H1 and H2 antagonists such as diphenhydramine (up to 50 mg IV) and ranitidine (1 mg/kg); steroids such as hydrocortisone 200 mg (IM or slow IV); nebulized beta-agonists; and crystalloid 500–1,000 ml IV.

Amniotic fluid embolism

Amniotic fluid embolism is a rare and largely unavoidable condition. It occurs when amniotic fluid enters the maternal circulation, causing maternal collapse, and often leads to cardiac arrest. A startling 5% of direct maternal deaths in the United States were attributed to this disorder (which may reflect the difficulty in making a definitive diagnosis).[4] The woman is often conscious at the onset of symptoms. Presentation is typically acute with shivering, sweating, anxiety, and coughing, followed by respiratory distress and cardiovascular collapse (hypotension, tachycardia, and possible arrhythmias). DIC may then quickly develop (within 20 to 60 minutes), causing massive maternal hemorrhage.

The diagnosis is initially presumptive and ultimately one of exclusion. Treatment involves support for the respiratory and cardiovascular systems and correction of clotting abnormalities.

If the woman survives, the identification of vernix, fetal hair, or fetal squames from the maternal right-sided circulation is supportive but not diagnostic. Fetal squames have been recovered in the maternal sputum in some cases. The presence of pulmonary hypertension may also be demonstrated.

Air embolism

An air embolism may occur following a ruptured uterus, during administration of intravenous fluids or blood products under pressure, or following manipulation of the placenta at cesarean section. Air embolism is associated with chest pain and collapse. An important differentiating factor from amniotic fluid embolism is auscultation with a stethoscope of an atypical millwheel murmur (or similarly distinguished with a fetal cardiotachometer) over the second right intercostal space.

References

1. Sentinel event alert issue 30: July 21, 2004. Preventing infant death and injury during delivery. *Adv Neonatal Care* 2004; 4: 180–1.

2. Lewis G (ed.) The Confidential Enquiry into Maternal and Child Health (CEMACH). *Saving Mothers' Lives: Reviewing Maternal Deaths to Make Motherhood Safer 2003–2005. The Seventh Report on Confidential Enquiries into Maternal Deaths in the United Kingdom*. London: CEMACH; 2007.

3. Knight M, Kenyon S, Brocklehurst P, Neilson J, Shakespeare J, Kurinczuk JJ (eds) on behalf of MBRRACEUK. *Saving Lives, Improving Mothers' Care: Lessons Learned to Inform Future Maternity Care from the UK and Ireland Confidential Enquiries into Maternal Deaths and Morbidity 2009–12*. Oxford: National Perinatal Epidemiology Unit, University of Oxford; 2014.

4. http://www.heart.org/idc/groups/heart-public/@wcm/@ecc/documents/downloadable/ucm_317350.pdf

5. Creanga AA, Berg CJ, Syverson C, Seed K, Bruce FC, Callaghan WM. Pregnancy-related mortality in the United States, 2006–2010. *Obstet Gynecol* 2015; 125: 5–12.

6. Virkus RA, Løkkegaard E, Lidegaard Ø, Langhoff-Roos J, Nielsen AK, Rothman KJ, Bergholt T. Risk factors for venous thromboembolism in 1.3 million pregnancies: a nationwide prospective cohort. *PLoS One* 2014; 9: e96495.

7. Oates S, Williams GL, Res GA. Cardiopulmonary resuscitation in late pregnancy. *Br Med J* 1988; 297: 404–5.

Module 3
Maternal cardiac arrest and advanced life support

Key learning points

- Management of cardiac arrest using the advanced cardiac life support (ACLS) algorithm.
- Review the causes of maternal cardiac arrest.
- Keep the woman supine during CPR and use manual left-uterine displacement on a firm surface (e.g., an operating table or resuscitation board) to reduce aortocaval compression.
- Perform/complete perimortem cesarean or instrumental delivery within 5 minutes of initiating resuscitation.
- Document the details of resuscitation: accurately, clearly, and legibly.

Common difficulties observed in training drills

- Focusing on ACLS to the exclusion of performing basic life support.
- Not manually displacing the uterus or performing closed chest massage on a firm surface.
- Not connecting the defibrillator.
- Stopping cardiac compressions as new staff arrive or while other actions are being performed.
- Not understanding perimortem cesarean section is performed primarily for maternal resuscitation.
- Forgetting to call the neonatal resuscitation team.

Introduction

Maternal cardiac arrest is rare and survival is low because the physiological changes of late pregnancy can hamper effective resuscitative efforts. The aim of this module is to provide obstetric staff with an overview of advanced life support as it relates to the pregnant woman. It is not intended to be a complete guide. More information and specific training is available elsewhere from credentialing bodies.[1,2]

Possible obstetric and anesthetic causes of cardiac arrest during pregnancy and postpartum include:

- hemorrhage
- pre-eclampsia/eclampsia
- pulmonary embolism
- amniotic fluid embolism
- septicemia
- total spinal anesthesia
- local anesthetic toxicity
- magnesium overdose.

These should be considered in addition to other causes of cardiac arrest in the non-pregnant woman (e.g., cardiac disease, substance abuse, anaphylaxis, trauma). Potentially reversible causes of cardiac arrest (the four Hs and the four Ts) are discussed later in this module.

Cardiorespiratory changes in pregnancy

The gravid uterus causes aortocaval compression when the woman is supine. At term, the inferior vena cava is completely occluded in 90% of supine women, resulting in up to a 70% decrease in cardiac stroke volume (the amount of blood pumped with each heart beat). Unaddressed, this compression significantly reduces the achievable cardiac output during cardiopulmonary resuscitation (CPR).

To ensure aortocaval compression is kept to a minimum while still maintaining good-quality, effective chest compressions, the woman should be kept supine with the uterus manually displaced to the left by an assistant using one or two hands (Figure 3.1).[3] Though not as efficient, but practical in a one- or two-rescuer situation, a woman on an operating table or another firm surface (e.g., a rescue board) can be tilted up to 30 degrees to the left.

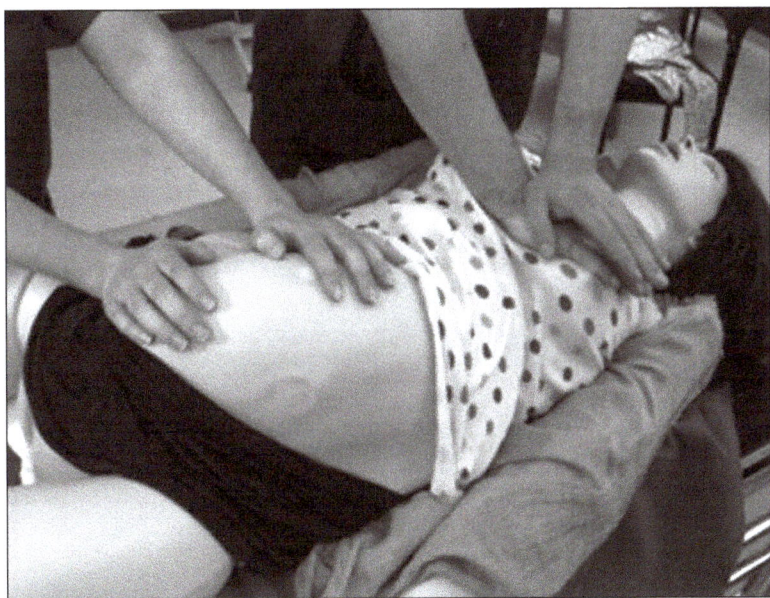

Figure 3.1 Manual displacement of the uterus to the left while administering CPR

Delivery should be expedited if the resuscitation is still unsuccessful after 4 minutes of effective CPR. An instrumental vaginal delivery can be performed if the woman is fully dilated and the baby is easily deliverable; otherwise, a perimortem cesarean section should be done. Emptying the uterus immediately relieves vena caval obstruction and significantly improves survival of the mother.[4,5,6] It may also improve survival rates for the infant but this is not the primary reason for undertaking the perimortem cesarean section.

The pregnant woman at term has a 20% decrease in functional residual lung capacity and a 20% increase in oxygen consumption. As a result, she becomes hypoxic more rapidly than the non-pregnant woman.[7] The enlarged uterus, together with the resulting upward displacement of the abdominal organs, decreases lung compliance during ventilation, which makes adequate mask ventilation during cardiac arrest even more difficult.

In addition, pregnancy increases the risk of aspiration of gastric contents; tracheal intubation reduces this risk. However, oxygenation of the patient always takes priority. Therefore prolonged attempts at tracheal intubation should be abandoned in favor of non-surgical (e.g., LMA) or surgical (e.g., cricothyrotomy) techniques.

Management of maternal cardiac arrest

An algorithm for the management of maternal cardiac arrest is shown in Figure 3.2. A more detailed list of the actions required in the event of maternal cardiac arrest is given in Box 3.1.

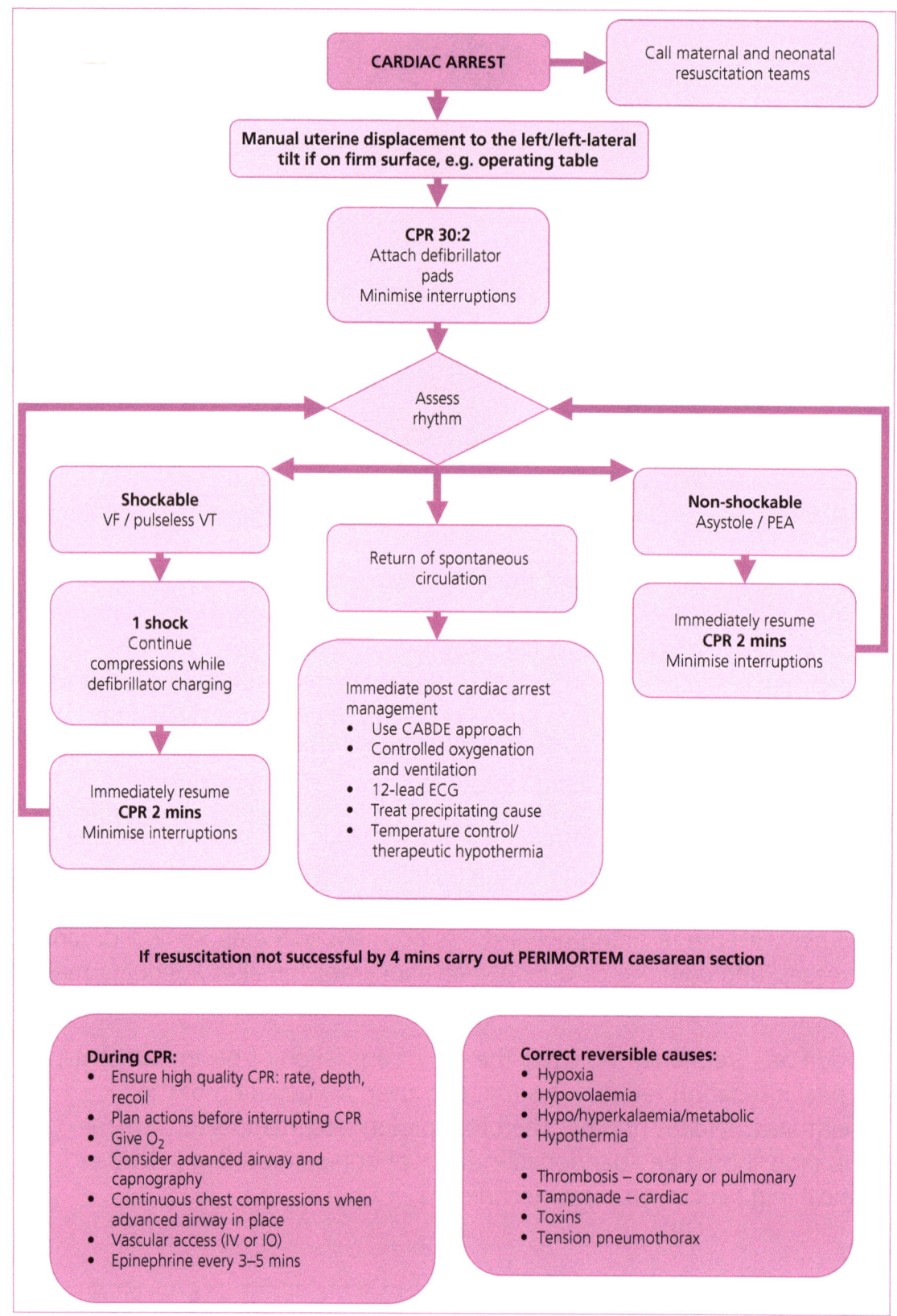

Figure 3.2 Adapted algorithm for the management of maternal cardiac arrest

Box 3.1 Management of maternal cardiac arrest

Event	Action
Help	■ Shout for help
	■ **Ring emergency number** and state "**maternal cardiac arrest**" and location of the incident
	■ Ask for the code cart including the defibrillator and perimortem cesarean section pack to be brought to the bedside
	■ **Call neonatal team (if the patient is still pregnant)**
	■ Inform unit security staff so the code team can enter the secured location without delay
	■ Contact the blood bank and ask for emergency blood products to be released
	■ Lay the bed flat
Positioning	■ Using clear, unambiguous language, calmly begin to delegate responsibilities as additional personnel arrive. Ask an assistant to manually displace the uterus to the left (and place a resuscitation board under the patient)
	■ Move the bed into the center of the room to allow adequate space for all personnel needed for maternal and fetal resuscitation
	■ Take the head end off the bed to allow access to the airway
Basic life support	■ Open airway
	■ Give 30 chest compressions (at rate of 100–120 compressions/minute) in middle of the sternum (more rostral than in a non-pregnant adult) to a depth of 5–6 cm: the emphasis is on good-quality chest compressions with regard to rate, depth, and recoil
	■ Next, give 2 breaths using a pocket mask or bag/mask ventilation
	■ Continue at ratio of 30 chest compressions to 2 breaths (each breath lasting 1 second)

Box 3.1 Management of maternal cardiac arrest (continued)

Event	Action
Equipment	■ **Defibrillator** – immediately apply gel pads and view rhythm to decide if a shock should be given: continue chest compressions while pads are applied
	■ Deliver shock if appropriate; CONTINUE chest compressions while defibrillator is charging or, if using an AED, follow instructions
	■ **Perimortem cesarean equipment** – open perimortem cesarean pack and disposable scalpel or instrumental set, and be ready to deliver baby by 5 minutes if CPR unsuccessful; alert OR team if appropriate
Investigations	■ **Large-bore IV access** should be obtained as soon as possible. Insertion of an interosseous needle is indicated should IV access be suboptimal
	■ **Venous blood** – send urgently for CBC, BUN, electrolytes, LFTs, clotting screen, cross-match, Ca^{2+}, and Mg^{2+}
	■ **Arterial blood gas** – some units may have blood gas analyzers that also provide hemoglobin, K^+, Na^+, Ca^{2+}, and glucose measurements in addition to the pH, PaO_2, and $PaCO_2$
Advanced life support	■ As soon as the code team arrives, a team leader should be appointed if not predetermined. Ideally, the team leader should coordinate the arrest, allocating specific tasks to members of the team but should not directly provide "hands-on" care required of ACLS.
	■ CPR should be uninterrupted, except for counter-shocks and rhythm checks (where appropriate), including during cesarean section, if required
	■ An anesthesiologist, if present, will normally manage the airway. If the anesthesiologist is the designated team leader, another anesthesiologist should be called to attend. Once the woman is

Box 3.1 Management of maternal cardiac arrest (continued)	
Event	**Action**
	intubated, chest compressions should be continuous. Capnography should be used if available
	■ **Shocks** – every 2 minutes if VF/pulseless VT
	■ **Epinephrine** – 1 mg IV flushed with at least 20 ml normal sterile saline for injections (after 3rd shock if VF/pulseless VT), repeated every 3–5 minutes. Vasopressin (40 U) can be substituted for one dose of epinephrine
Deliver the baby	■ If resuscitation has not succeeded within 5 minutes, then deliver by quickest means (cesarean section or forceps); this means the obstetric team is prompted 4 minutes into the resuscitation by the person assigned to keep time
	■ Continue CPR during operation
	■ Ensure the neonatal team is in attendance
Documentation	■ Note the time of the arrest (if witnessed), arrival of staff, timing of defibrillation, timing of drugs administered, time of delivery, and time cardiac output is regained

Role of the team leader

The team leader is usually a physician on the code team; however, it could be anybody trained in advanced life support. In the operating room, the team leader would be the anesthesiologist. The team leader should direct the team and ensure their safety. This is best achieved by standing back, delegating specific tasks to members of the team, and ensuring that clear commands are given. The team leader must consider any correctable cause of cardiac arrest and decide whether administering any other drugs (Table 3.1) may be beneficial.

In a maternal cardiac arrest, it is important the team leader (or any other member of the team) state immediately after arrest occurs that a perimortem delivery (by cesarean section unless the woman is fully dilated) will need to be

Table 3.1 Drugs to be considered during cardiac arrest

Feature	Drug to be considered
Cardiac arrest	1 mg epinephrine IV every 3–5 minutes
VF/VT	300 mg amiodarone IV after third counter-shock
Opiate overdose	0.4–0.8 mg naloxone IV
Magnesium toxicity	1 g calcium gluconate IV (or, 333 mg calcium chloride IV)
Bupivacaine toxicity	1.5 ml/kg intralipid 20% IV initial bolus

The tracheal route is not recommended. Drugs should be administered via the intravenous or intraosseous route.

performed within 5 minutes of initiating CPR if resuscitation is unsuccessful. Hence the team must be ready to start 3–4 minutes into the resuscitation. The equipment necessary should be immediately prepared (Figure 3.3). Someone not directly providing hands-on care during the resuscitation should keep a written record of the time from initiation. It is important the neonatal team be called as soon as a maternal arrest is discovered so they have time to prepare the equipment required for neonatal resuscitation.

> **It is important to continue with CPR throughout the cesarean or instrumental delivery.**

The code team leader should decide when a resuscitation attempt should be abandoned, typically done in consultation with the rest of the team. The team leader is responsible for documenting the arrest.

It is good practice to ensure someone remains with the relatives during an arrest and keeps them as informed as possible. After the arrest, support for the family should be immediately available, as well as separate efforts made to support the personnel involved in the management of the unfortunate patient. As important, and perhaps an even more delicate procedure, a medical "de-brief" should be scheduled by the unit/institution at a time convenient to all involved in the arrest.

Recognition of heart rhythms

Resuscitation attempts should follow the evidence-based algorithms published by the American Heart Association.[1] The advanced life support algorithm (Figure 3.2) has two main pathways, and the cardiac rhythm dictates which pathway to follow: those requiring direct current cardioversion ("shockable

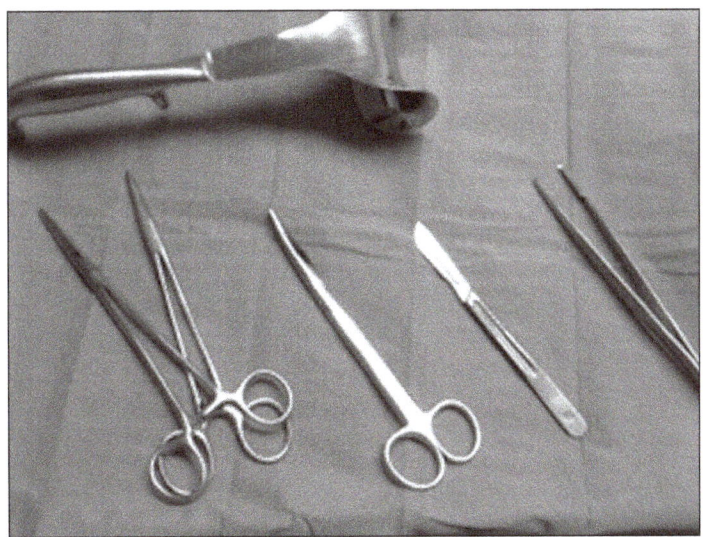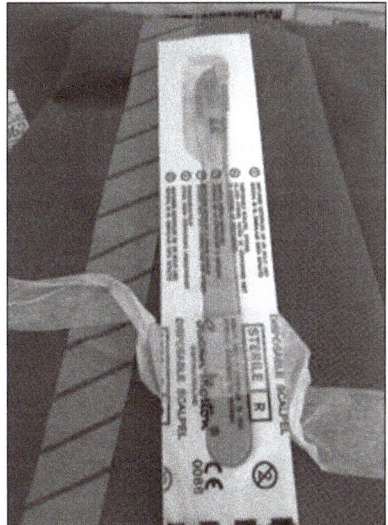

Figure 3.3 Equipment required for perimortem cesarean section, with disposable scalpel attached to outside of pack

Box 3.2 Heart rhythms found during cardiac arrest	
Shockable rhythms	**Non-shockable rhythms**
Ventricular fibrillation (VF)	Asystole
Pulseless ventricular tachycardia (VT)	Pulseless electrical activity (PEA)

rhythms") and those in which cardioversion would be inappropriate ("non-shockable rhythms") (Box 3.2).

Once cardiac arrest is confirmed, a defibrillator should be used to rapidly assess the cardiac rhythm. Self-adhesive pads are placed on the woman's chest and may be used for both cardiac monitoring and/or defibrillation. *Do not stop chest compressions to apply the pads.*

The EKG leads are color coded and should be attached with the red electrode to the right shoulder (Red to Right), the yellow electrode to the left shoulder (yeLLow to Left), and the green electrode below the pectoral muscles (green for spleen) (Figure 3.4). The defibrillator should be altered to read the EKG rhythm through lead two. Alternatively, the cardiac rhythm may be viewed through the self-adhesive defibrillator pads attached to the woman's chest, as illustrated in Figure 3.4.

During arrest, the heart rhythms seen will fit into one of the two categories: shockable or non-shockable (Box 3.2).

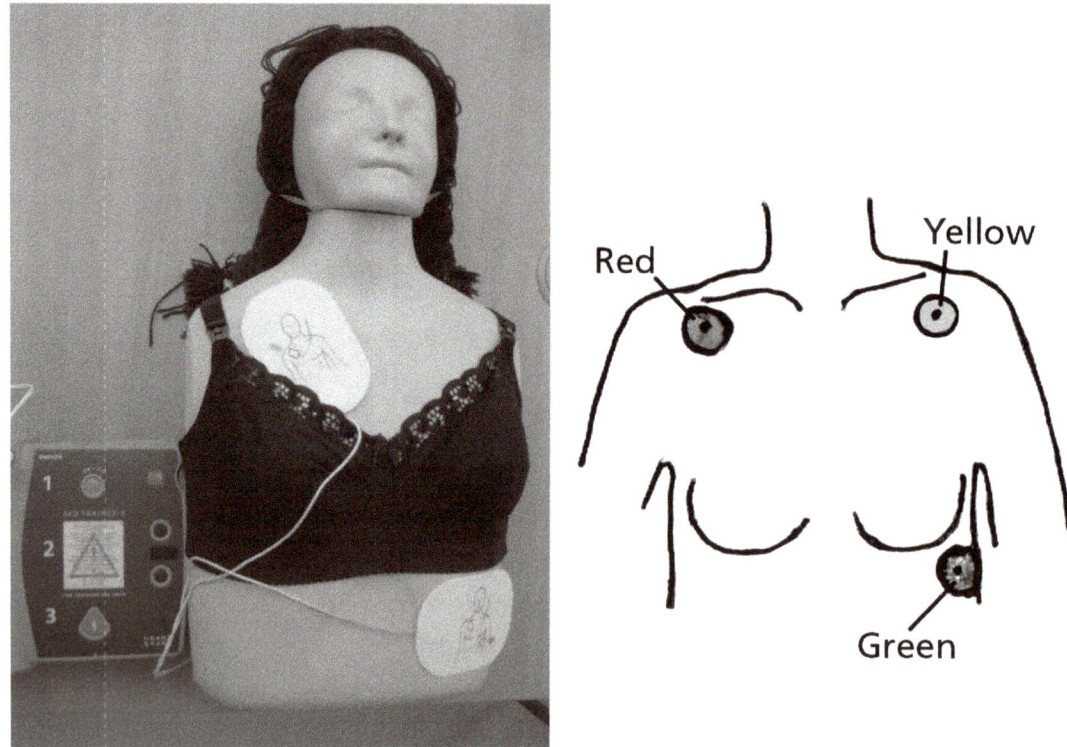

Figure 3.4 Defibrillation pads and EKG electrode placement

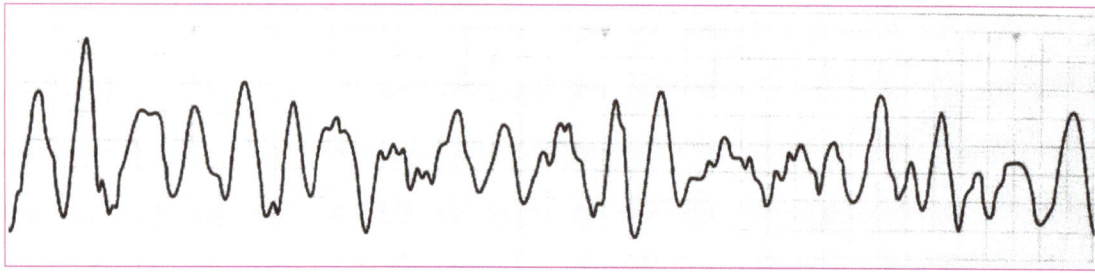

Figure 3.5 An example of ventricular fibrillation (VF)

Shockable rhythms

The majority of survivors from cardiac arrests are in the shockable rhythm category (VF and pulseless VT). A typical example of VF is shown in Figure 3.5.

VT is characterized by a broad-complex regular tachycardia (Figure 3.6). VT can cause a profound loss of cardiac output and can suddenly deteriorate into VF. Pulseless VT is treated in the same way as VF.

Shockable cardiac rhythms require defibrillation: the passing of an electrical current across the heart to simultaneously depolarize a critical mass of myocardium so that the natural pacemaking tissue of the heart can resume control. *Attempted defibrillation is the single most important step in the*

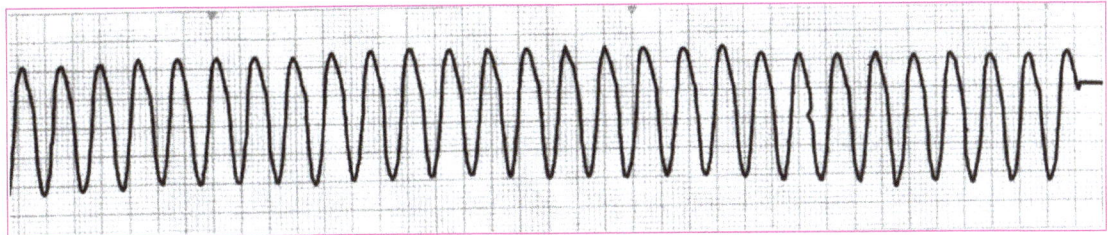

Figure 3.6 Ventricular tachycardia (VT)

treatment of VF/VT. The time between the onset of VF/VT and defibrillation is the main determinant of patient survival. **Survival falls by 7–10% for each minute following collapse.**

Most defibrillators now transmit a biphasic current, which has a higher efficiency, so less energy is required to depolarize the heart. When using a biphasic defibrillator, a current of 150–200 joules (J) should be used for the first shock, and 150–360 J for subsequent shocks; for a monophasic defibrillator, 360 J should be used for the first and subsequent shocks.

> **Know your machine: if unsure, shock at 200 J.**

Remember: only one shock per cycle is given for shockable rhythms; the shock is then immediately followed by 2 minutes of CPR at a ratio of 30 compressions to 2 ventilations (without checking for a rhythm or a pulse). After 2 minutes, the rhythm should be checked and a second shock delivered, if required. A pulse should be checked only if a non-shockable rhythm is seen.

> **Epinephrine 1 mg IV should be given after alternate shocks (every 3–5 minutes, starting immediately after the third shock).**
>
> **Amiodarone 300 mg IV should be given after the third shock.**

Most clinical areas now have automated external defibrillators (AEDs), which are able to analyze the cardiac rhythm and deliver an appropriate shock if indicated. It is important to continue chest compressions while the defibrillator is charging, prior to the delivery of the shock. If using an AED, follow the machine's instructions. Figure 3.7 shows an example of an AED used for training.

Non-shockable rhythms

Pulseless electrical activity (PEA) is the clinical absence of cardiac output (i.e., no pulse) despite cardiac electrical activity, which may be interpreted as normal

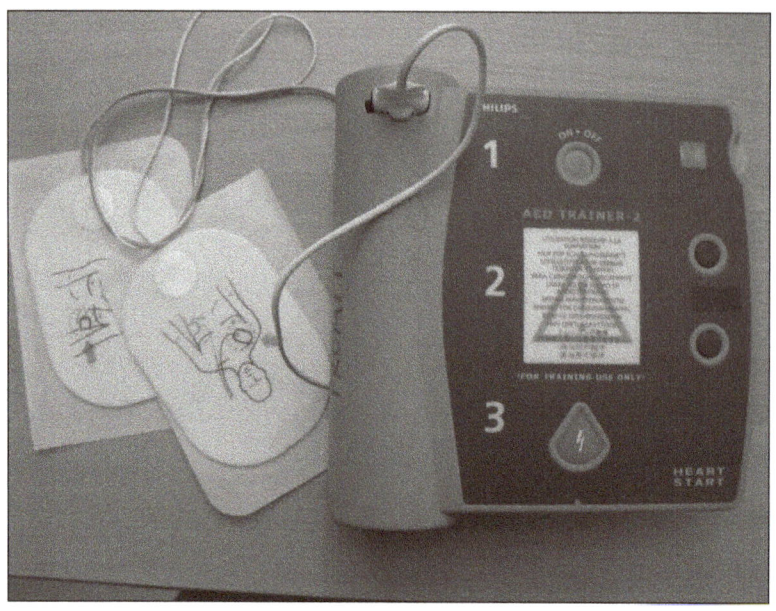

Figure 3.7 An example of an AED machine used for training

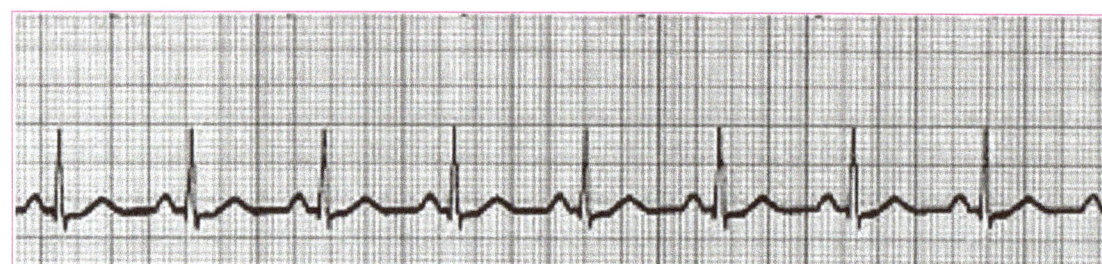

Figure 3.8 Normal sinus rhythm or electrical activity that can be found in pulseless electrical activity

(or near-normal) sinus rhythm. For example, in exsanguination, the heart's electrical activity may continue to show a normal sinus rhythm, as shown in Figure 3.8, yet there is no circulating blood so a pulse is not present.

Asystole is a slightly wandering flat line; an example is shown in Figure 3.9. *Until proven otherwise, a COMPLETELY flat horizontal line indicates that the monitoring leads are not correctly attached rather than asystole. Adults in asystole have a very poor prognosis. Asystole is NOT a shockable rhythm.*

- **If there is any doubt about whether the rhythm is asystole or fine VF, do not attempt defibrillation; instead, continue chest compressions and ventilation 30:2.**

- **Epinephrine 1 mg IV should be given as soon as possible and then every 3–5 minutes.**

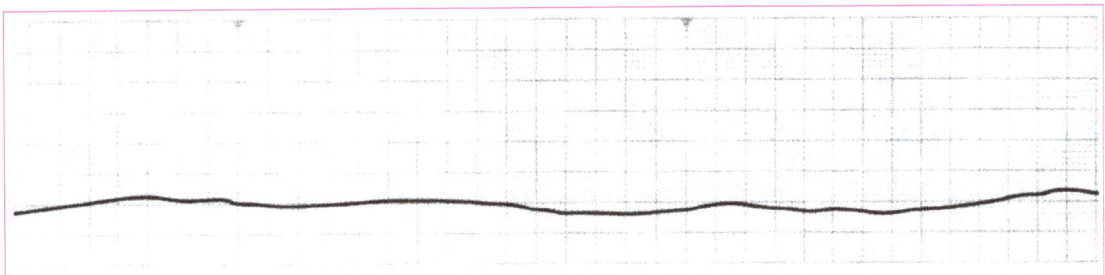

Figure 3.9 Asystole

Potentially reversible causes

If the cardiac rhythm is not VF or VT, the outcome will be poor unless a potentially reversible cause can be found and treated. Potentially reversible causes of cardiac arrest can be remembered using the four "Hs" and four "Ts."

The four Hs

1. **Hypoxia** – ensure the patient is adequately ventilated during the arrest. Basic life support followed by prompt, effective airway management (intubation, non-surgical, or surgical airways) with adequate ventilation using 100% oxygen should maximize oxygen delivery to the woman. Check for chest rise and bilateral air entry during ventilation.

2. **Hypovolemia** is most commonly caused by massive hemorrhage (such as abruption or postpartum hemorrhage). Start intravenous fluids and blood products promptly to restore the intravascular volume; consider emergent surgical intervention to correct the cause of bleeding if not amenable to non-invasive approaches.

3. **Hypo-/hyperkalemia/metabolic**

   ■ **Hypoglycemia** may occur in a diabetic mother. If the blood glucose measures below 55 mg/dl (3 mmol/l), give 50 ml of 25% glucose solution IV.

   ■ **Hyperkalemia** (high serum potassium) can develop secondary to renal failure.

   ■ **Hypermagnesemia** (high serum magnesium) may result from treatment of pre-eclampsia with intravenous magnesium sulfate, especially with concurrent renal impairment. Magnesium should not be used for the treatment of preterm labor for which it is ineffective.

   ■ **Hypocalcemia** (low serum calcium) can result from overdose of calcium channel blocking drugs such as nifedipine.

High serum levels of potassium or magnesium and low serum levels of calcium should be treated with 1 g of calcium gluconate (10 ml of 10%) IV.

4. **Hypothermia** is an unlikely cause of in-hospital maternal arrest but is often seen complicating the arrest of a previously laboring, unclothed patient. Keep the patient warm in the peri-arrest situation by using warmed intravenous fluids and warming blankets when appropriate. However, once a cardiac arrest has occurred, there is evidence that mild therapeutic hypothermia (to 35 degrees) can actually provide neuroprotection.[8]

The four Ts

1. **Thromboemboli** are more common in pregnancy owing to the procoagulant effect of pregnancy and the mechanical obstruction of venous return by the gravid uterus. Massive pulmonary embolus can cause sudden collapse and cardiac arrest. Treatment is difficult but thrombolysis, cardiopulmonary bypass, or operative removal of the clot should be considered. Amniotic fluid emboli are also a cause of sudden collapse and cardiac arrest. Treatment remains supportive and care should be taken to correct clotting abnormalities as disseminated intravascular coagulopathy often results. Early consultation with a hematologist should be considered considering the prospect of massive transfusion and potentially a need for anti-fibrinolytics or other drugs.

2. **Tension pneumothorax** can cause collapse and subsequent PEA. A tension pneumothorax is most likely to occur during trauma. However, it can occur during resuscitation after an attempted insertion of a central venous catheter or after closed chest compressions. Treatment requires acute decompression of the affected side by inserting a large peripheral intravenous cannula into the thoracic cavity in the second intercostal space at the midclavicular line, followed by chest drain insertion.

3. **Therapeutic** or **toxic** substances (for example, inadvertent administration of bupivacaine intravenously or opiate overdose) can cause arrest. Specific anti-dotes or treatments should be used; for an opiate overdose, naloxone 0.4–0.8 mg IV or, for bupivacaine overdose, intralipid 1.5 ml/kg IV, followed either by repeat bolus, if unstable, or continuous infusion (15 ml/kg/hour), if stable.

4. Cardiac **tamponade** is an uncommon cause of maternal arrest but should be considered after trauma, especially when there are penetrating chest injuries. Tamponade is corrected by pericardiocentesis.

Drugs used during cardiac arrest

Epinephrine 1 mg should be given IV every 3–5 minutes during a cardiac arrest. Other drugs that may be considered are listed in Table 3.1.

All drugs should be flushed with at least 20 ml saline to ensure they enter the central circulation. The most common drugs required for a cardiac arrest are kept on the code cart in prefilled syringes, so that they can be quickly administered in an emergency. It is important that all staff members are aware of the location of the code cart and defibrillator on their unit. It is also important that staff familiarize themselves with the use of their local emergency equipment and drugs, as equipment may vary between locations.

Post-resuscitation care

A comprehensive, structured post-resuscitation protocol is important and would normally include transfer to an intensive care unit:

- CABDE approach.
- Controlled oxygenation and ventilation. Avoid hyperoxia. The inspired oxygen should be titrated to maintain arterial oxygen saturations at 94–98% (guided by a pulse oximeter or arterial blood gas).
- Temperature and glucose control should be addressed using institutional guidelines. Therapeutic hypothermia should be considered. Glucose levels greater than 180 mg/dl (10 mmol/l) should be treated but hypoglycemia avoided.
- A 12-lead EKG should be performed.
- Precipitating causes should be treated.

References

1. Neumar RW, Otto CW, Link MS, Kronick SL, Shuster M, Callaway CW, et al. Part 8: Adult advanced cardiovascular life support: 2010 American Heart Association Guidelines for Cardiopulmonary Resuscitation and Emergency Cardiovascular Care. *Circulation* 2010; 122 (suppl 3): S729–67.
2. Resuscitation Council (UK) [www.resus.org.uk].
3. Resuscitation Council (UK). FAQs on advanced life support. 2012 [www.resus.org.uk/page/faqALS.htm].
4. Marx G. Cardiopulmonary resuscitation of late-pregnant women. *Anaesthesiology* 1982; 56: 156.
5. Oates S, Williams GL, Res GA. Cardiopulmonary resuscitation in late pregnancy. *Br Med J* 1988; 297: 404–5.
6. Page-Rodriguez A, Gonzalez-Sanchez JA. Perimortem caesarean section of twin pregnancy: case report and review of the literature. *Acad Emerg Med* 1999; 6: 1072–4.
7. Zakowski MI, Ramanathan S. CPR in pregnancy. *Curr Rev Clin Anesth* 1990; 10: 106.
8. Arrich J, Holzer M, Herkner H, Müllner M. Hypothermia for neuroprotection in adults after cardiopulmonary resuscitation. *Cochrane Database Syst Rev* 2009; 4: CD004128.

Module 4
Maternal anesthetic emergencies

Key learning points

- Understand the potential difficulties in tracheal intubation of the obstetric patient.
- Understand the management of failed tracheal intubation.
- Recognition and management of high regional block.
- Signs and symptoms of local anesthetic toxicity.
- Management of cardiac arrest in a patient with local anesthetic toxicity.

Background

Though the percentage has been declining since 1986, anesthetic complications continue to be a direct cause of 0.7% of all maternal deaths in the United States.[1] In the Confidential Enquiry into Maternal Deaths in the United Kingdom 2006–08, half the women who died from either direct or indirect pregnancy causes had been administered an anesthetic agent. Of the 127 direct maternal deaths, 7 (3%) were attributed to anesthesia,[2] a slight increase in the rate over the previous triennium (0.31/100,000 maternities). Sadly, the care was judged substandard in 6 cases. There were a further 18 direct or indirect deaths in which perioperative or anesthesia management contributed, and another 12 cases of severe pre-eclampsia or sepsis where obstetricians or gynecologists failed to consult with either anesthesia or critical care services sufficiently early.[2] During a more recent period, MBRRACE observed that of the 82 direct maternal deaths, 4 were attributed to anesthetic causes. And although the anesthetic-related death rate had declined, the deaths involving anesthesia were invariably multi-factorial suggesting an opportunity for there to be lessons learned.[3]

The role of the anesthesiologist in the multi-disciplinary team involves unique challenges: their specific skills are often required in high-stress situations when time is critical and maternal or fetal life is at risk. It is in these circumstances that help from the rest of the maternity team can be invaluable.

Failed tracheal intubation

Introduction

General anesthesia for cesarean section is now uncommon. Box 4.1 lists the common indications for general anesthesia. Of the 157,359 cesarean sections performed in England and Wales from 2009 through 2010, less than 5% were performed under general anesthesia. The vast majority of general anesthetics were performed for emergencies (84.4%).[4]

The majority of complications due to general anesthesia relate to the airway. When the airway needs to be secured in a pregnant woman, it is important that a cuffed tracheal tube be inserted through and secured below the vocal cords to maintain a patent airway, as pregnant women are at increased risk of stomach regurgitation and aspiration.

The aspiration of gastric contents is sometimes fatal, but the failure to oxygenate is always fatal. Therefore a failed intubation is an anesthetic emergency. In the obstetric patient, a useful definition of a failed tracheal intubation is that it occurs after two failed attempts at tracheal intubation. It is then the failed intubation drill should begin, although it would be prudent to prepare to assist the anesthesiologist after the first failed attempt.

For several reasons, failed tracheal intubation in the obstetric patient is almost 10 times more common than in the general surgical population

---

Box 4.1 Indications for general anesthesia

- Severe maternal or fetal compromise requiring immediate delivery
- Regional anesthesia contraindicated (e.g., coagulopathy, hemodynamic or respiratory instability)
- Failed regional anesthesia
- Maternal request

Box 4.2 Risk factors for difficult intubation

- Known previous difficult intubation
- Obesity
- Pre-eclampsia
- Congenital airway difficulties with restricted neck movement and limited mouth opening (e.g., Klippel–Feil syndrome, Pierre Robin syndrome)
- Acquired airway difficulties with restricted neck movement and limited mouth opening (e.g., rheumatoid arthritis, ankylosing spondylitis, cervical spine fusions)

(1 in 250 compared with 1 in 2,200 in general surgical patients); reasons include: abnormal dentition, increased pharyngeal/laryngeal edema (especially in the edematous pre-eclamptic or even a routine patient who has been pushing in the second stage), and the larger tongue and breasts associated with pregnancy. In addition, pregnant women desaturate rapidly owing to the additional oxygen requirements of pregnancy.[5] The growing incidence of morbid obesity in pregnant women is also likely to increase the incidence of difficult tracheal intubation.

Ideally, all difficult intubations would be predicted antenatally. All women at risk of a difficult intubation could then be referred to the obstetric anesthesiologist (Box 4.2).

Unfortunately, individual screening tests used to identify patients with potentially difficult airways are unreliable – particularly in the obstetric population. As a result, the anesthesiologist may be faced with an unexpectedly difficult or impossible tracheal intubation. In such circumstances, it helps to use a clear algorithm to minimize the occurrence of any complications.

Management and reduction of potential complications

The management of failed tracheal intubation in the obstetric patient should involve early recognition of the potentially difficult airway. In such patients (such as morbidly obese mothers) some clinicians recommend inserting an epidural or spinal catheter early in labor.[6] This allows the option of injecting the catheter should an emergency cesarean become necessary. Otherwise, insertion of a spinal would be technically difficult at this time, and perhaps impossible, given the time constraints characteristic of an emergency cesarean section.

Gastric aspiration is more likely during a difficult intubation, in emergency cases, and in obese pregnant women. For this reason, particular attention should be paid to reducing the volume and acidity of the stomach contents in laboring high-risk women. Local guidelines should be created for high-risk women (e.g., morbid obesity, diabetic gastroparesis). For example, ingestion of isotonic liquids allowed in a routine labor might be discouraged in some patients deemed at high risk for difficult tracheal intubation. Regular prophylactic H_2 receptor antagonists might be given (e.g., oral or intravenous ranitidine in addition to the ingestion of antacid (e.g., sodium citrate) as commonly used before induction of obstetric anesthesia. These preventative measures provide another safeguard to reduce the potential morbidity and mortality associated with emergency obstetric surgery and anesthesia.

In the event of an emergency general anesthetic, adequate preparation before laryngoscopy may be the difference between success and failure at tracheal intubation. Optimal positioning of the mother is particularly important in morbidly obese women. Positioning on the table should ensure that the mother's head is as close to the anesthesiologist as possible, with pillows placed so that her neck is flexed and her chin pointing up towards the ceiling (Figure 4.1). This may require time to reposition the patient and the table after the obstetrician has failed to achieve a vaginal delivery in a patient whose legs were in stirrups.

It can be useful to adopt the "ramped" position in pregnant women, especially those with large breasts or who are obese, which has been shown to improve

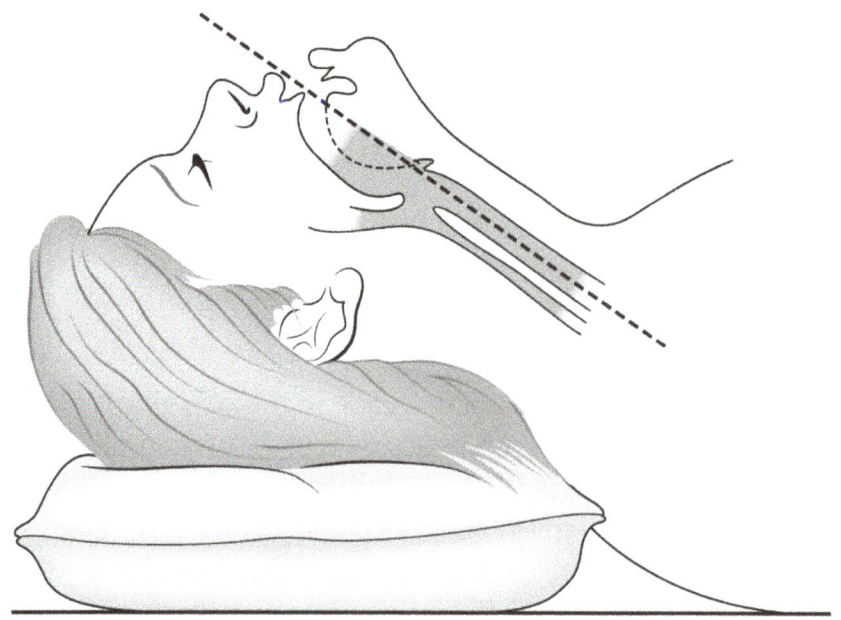

Figure 4.1 Optimal anatomical position for successful laryngoscopy

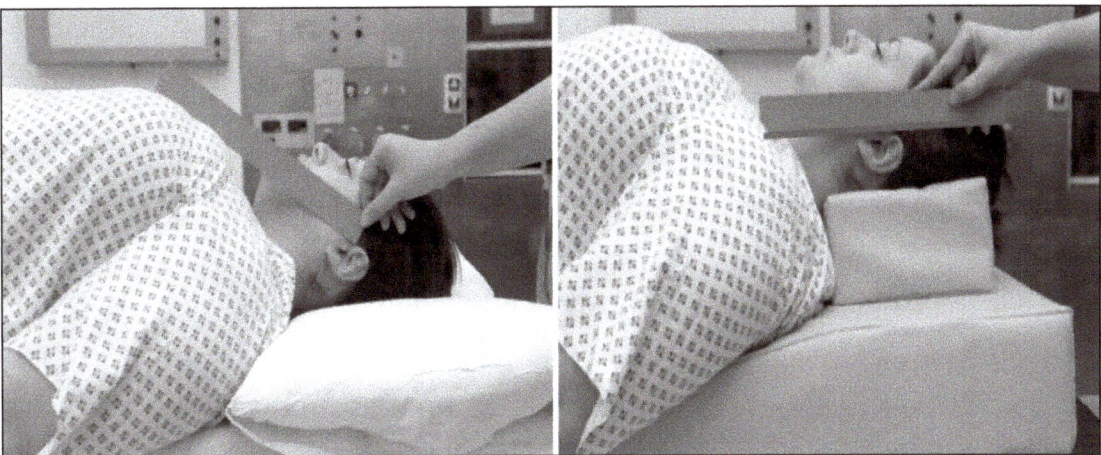

Figure 4.2 Anatomical realignment using the Oxford HELP to improve intubating conditions (©Alma Medical Products 2010, reproduced with permission)

the view of the vocal cords at laryngoscopy.[7] The ramped position seeks a horizontal line between the sternal notch and the external auditory meatus, as shown in Figure 4.2. The position can be achieved using purpose-made pillows such as the Oxford HELP (head elevating laryngoscopy pillow) or by adjusting the operating table and using extra pillows and wedges.

Pre-oxygenation should begin once the woman is positioned on the operating table. Pre-oxygenation is important to prevent desaturation, which can occur rapidly during intubation in pregnant women. The aim is to fill the lungs with as much oxygen as possible while removing nitrogen, so that upon induction of anesthesia, when the patient has stopped breathing, there is enough oxygen available for gaseous exchange during laryngoscopy, tracheal intubation, and initiation of mechanical ventilation. For effective pre-oxygenation, the "anesthesia" facemask must be tightly applied to the patient's face, not leaving any room for air (mostly nitrogen) to enter and dilute the oxygen delivered by the anesthesia machine. At this stage, the team can help by attaching monitor equipment and preparing the abdomen and drapes, allowing the anesthesiologist to begin immediate pre-oxygenation minimizing the time to induction of general anesthesia, skin incision, and delivery.

It is important for the operating room (OR) team to remain quiet during the induction of anesthesia, and to be prepared to help in the event of a failed intubation. If tracheal intubation does fail, then the anesthesiologist should immediately declare the emergency, stating "this is a failed intubation." Individual roles will vary during this emergency. The anesthesiologist and obstetrician are unable to leave the woman, so other team members will need to provide assistance. All OR staff should know where the "difficult airway equipment" is kept and be able to retrieve it, if requested. All OR staff should also know how to call for additional personnel (e.g., anesthetic assistants, head and neck surgeons) and equipment to assist the anesthesiologist. A failed intubation is a very stressful situation; clear communication is essential.

The failed intubation algorithm is outlined in Figure 4.3.

In the event of a failed intubation, the life of the woman is the anesthesiologist's priority. The patient is classified as either "can ventilate/oxygenate" or "cannot ventilate/oxygenate." In most instances, the woman who can be ventilated/oxygenated must be awakened, but, in exceptional circumstances, it may be appropriate to continue with surgery. Under these circumstances, the procedure will be performed under a non-routine general anesthetic, the woman spontaneously breathing high concentrations of anesthetic gas via anesthetic mask or some type of supraglottic device (e.g., laryngeal mask airway (LMA)) without muscle relaxation. The cesarean section will be technically more difficult for the surgeon, as gaining access to the uterus can be problematic without abdominal relaxation and the high concentrations of anesthetic gases may cause uterine relaxation and increase the risk of hemorrhage. It is important that the most senior obstetrician performs the surgery as quickly as possible to limit the duration of surgery. An anesthetized pregnant patient can "lose" their non-intubated airway at any time, quickly leading to disaster.

Box 4.3 outlines best practice points for tracheal intubation.

Box 4.3 Best practice points for tracheal intubation

- Identify women at risk and refer for antenatal anesthetic assessment
- Assess the airway before induction of anesthesia
- Anesthesiologists should check all intubation and difficult airway equipment daily and be familiar with its use and location
- Position the patient correctly before induction
- Pre-oxygenate carefully
- Call for help early
- Remember that oxygenation is more important than intubation

---

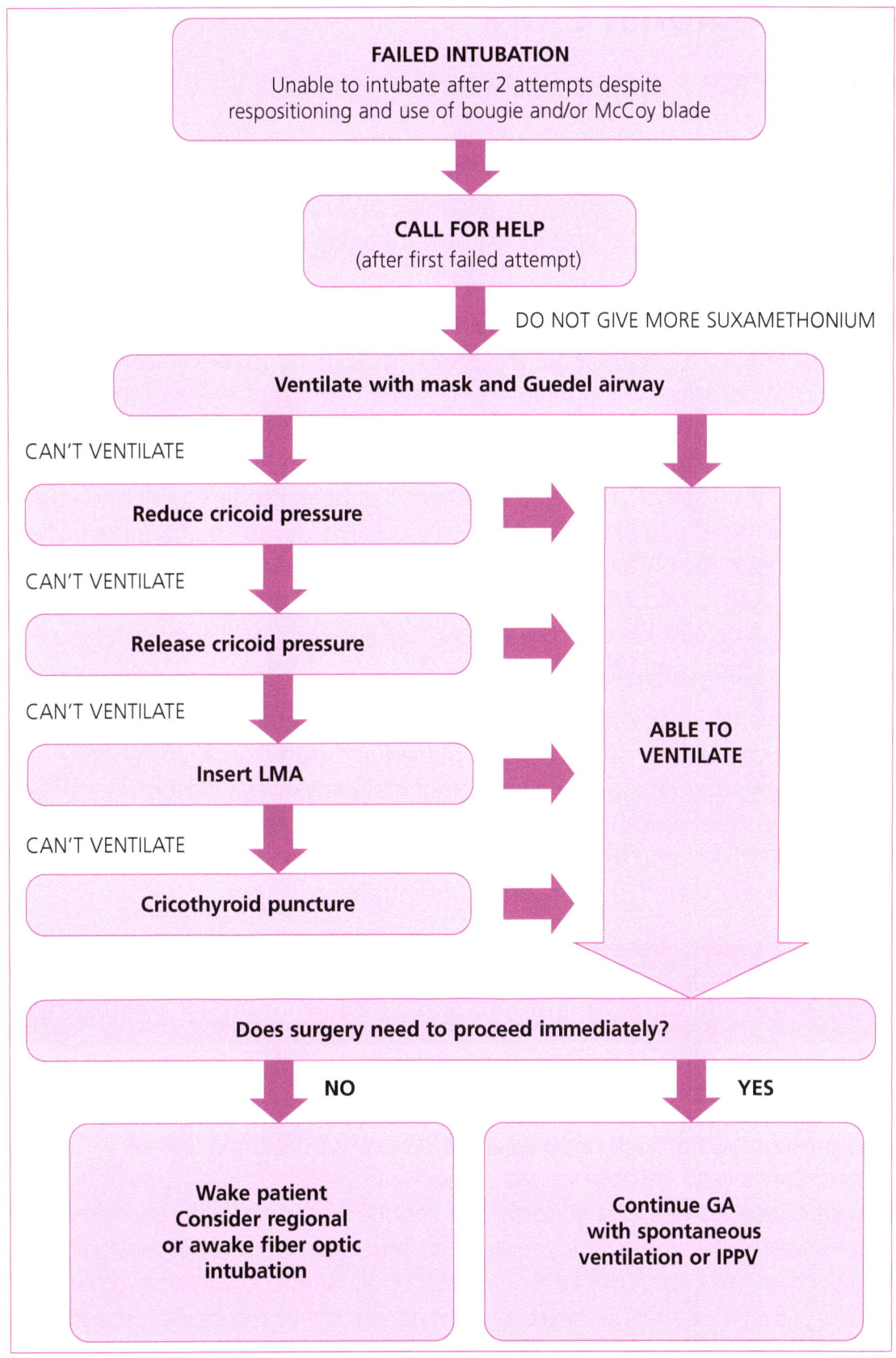

Figure 4.3 Algorithm for management of failed intubation[8]

High regional block

Introduction

A high block after spinal or epidural anesthesia that requires the patient be intubated has been described as "the failed intubation of the new millennium."[9] This is because the incidence of a high regional block has increased as regional anesthesia has gradually replaced non-emergent general anesthesia.

The height of the block following spinal or epidural anesthesia varies among patients. The term "high block" encompasses a spectrum of clinical events. At one end of the spectrum, a patient may have mild symptoms and require only reassurance with or without supplemental oxygen; at the other end of the spectrum, the patient may stop breathing, which can lead to cardiac arrest. The term "total spinal" implies the patient has been rendered unconscious. Total spinal is defined as cardiorespiratory collapse caused by the direct action of local anesthetic on the high cervical nerve roots and brainstem. While caution is used in calculating spinal anesthesia doses, the specter of total spinal must always be considered. Fortunately, it is a rare complication of epidural anesthesia (approximately 1 in 16,000).[10,11]

A high regional block can occur inadvertently in several ways. It can be an exaggerated response to correctly placed and dosed local anesthetic, the result of an unintentional overdose of local anesthetic during spinal or epidural anesthesia, or the result of an unintentional injection of local anesthetic into the wrong space (e.g., injection of an epidural catheter unintentionally seated in the subdural or intrathecal space).

> **Both total spinal and high block with inadequate breathing requiring intubation are anesthetic emergencies.**

Presentation

The presentation of high regional block can vary from rapid loss of consciousness and collapse to a gradual rise in the block level with or without loss of consciousness. It is important to monitor pregnant women closely after spinal and epidural anesthesia. High block can occur after any epidural top-up dose and especially while dosing rapidly before emergency cesarean delivery. Everyone must be alert to warning signs that the block is extending above the desired level (Box 4.4).

Especially after spinal anesthesia, some women will have a block that reaches the lower cervical nerve roots. Diaphragmatic breathing is not compromised,

Box 4.4 Warning signs of rising block

- Nausea
- "Not feeling right"
- Breathlessness
- Tingling fingers or arms
- Difficulty speaking
- Difficulty swallowing
- Sedation

Box 4.5 Risk factors for high regional block

- Unintentional dural puncture (recognized or unrecognized) during epidural insertion
- Unintentional subdural placement of epidural catheter (subdural catheters can migrate into the subarachnoid space)
- Large or rapid epidural top-ups (e.g., as seen before an emergent cesarean section)
- Spinal injection after the in situ epidural is deemed inadequate for anesthesia
- Epidural dose to reinforce inadequate spinal anesthesia (combined spinal–epidural)

but the women often complain they "can't breathe." Reassurance may suffice, but it is still important to call for help, watch the woman closely, assess her pulse, blood pressure, respiratory rate, and oxygen saturations, and look for the warning signs outlined in Box 4.4.

If the local anesthetic reaches the upper cervical nerve roots, blocking the nerves supplying the diaphragm, the woman will not be able to adequately ventilate and will rapidly become hypoxic. If the brainstem is affected (total spinal), there is likely to be severe hypotension and bradycardia. Fetal bradycardia may occur as a result of reduced placental blood flow and/or maternal hypoxia.

There are several risk factors for high regional block, which mean it is not a complication confined to the operating room (Box 4.5). High regional block should be in the differential diagnosis of maternal collapse in any woman receiving an epidural.

Management

In the situation where a woman shows warning signs of a high block (Box 4.4), it is imperative to remain with her and to call for help early in case she continues to deteriorate (Figure 4.4).

The emergency call system should be used to immediately summon help in the event of a total spinal characterized by cardiorespiratory collapse or a high block with inadequate ventilation. It may be necessary to call the cardiac arrest team to

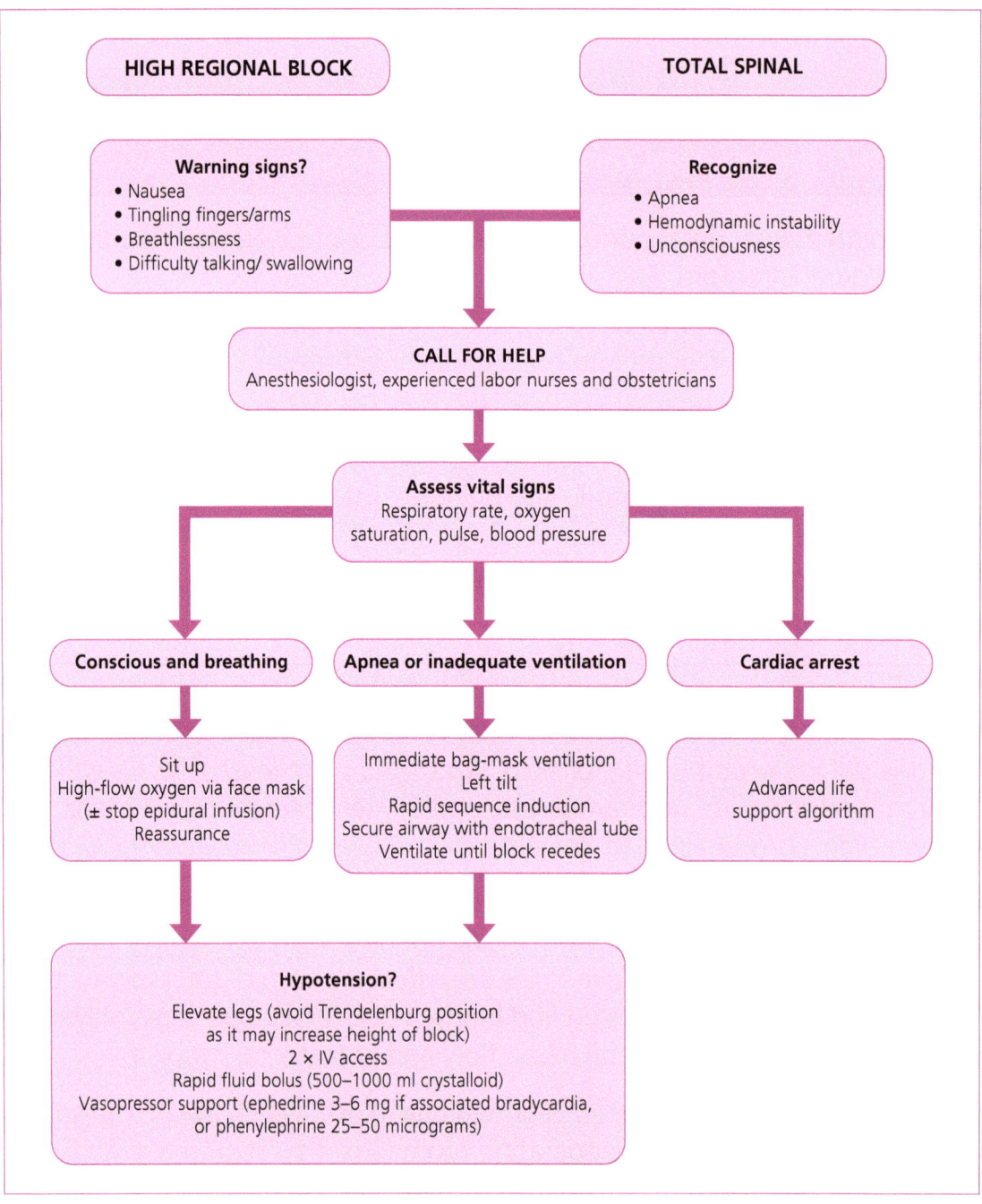

HIGH REGIONAL BLOCK

TOTAL SPINAL

Warning signs?
- Nausea
- Tingling fingers/arms
- Breathlessness
- Difficulty talking/ swallowing

Recognize
- Apnea
- Hemodynamic instability
- Unconsciousness

CALL FOR HELP
Anesthesiologist, experienced labor nurses and obstetricians

Assess vital signs
Respiratory rate, oxygen saturation, pulse, blood pressure

Conscious and breathing

Apnea or inadequate ventilation

Cardiac arrest

Sit up
High-flow oxygen via face mask
(± stop epidural infusion)
Reassurance

Immediate bag-mask ventilation
Left tilt
Rapid sequence induction
Secure airway with endotracheal tube
Ventilate until block recedes

Advanced life
support algorithm

Hypotension?

Elevate legs (avoid Trendelenburg position
as it may increase height of block)
2 × IV access
Rapid fluid bolus (500–1000 ml crystalloid)
Vasopressor support (ephedrine 3–6 mg if associated bradycardia,
or phenylephrine 25–50 micrograms)

Figure 4.4 Management algorithm for high regional block

ensure that enough skilled people are present to simultaneously intubate the woman, manage ventilation and circulatory support, expedite delivery, and give advanced life support if cardiac arrest ensues (see Module 2 and Module 3).

Remember: call for help, assess CAB and deliver 100% oxygen.

The woman should immediately be mask ventilated while the airway equipment is prepared for tracheal intubation. Circulatory support, in the form of intravenous fluids, vasopressors, and inotropes will be necessary, particularly if there is a total spinal. Maternal hypotension, (inadequate cardiac filling) leads to bradycardia just before cardiac arrest, in which case chest compressions should be initiated immediately on a rescue board (with manual left-uterine displacement) and advanced life support instituted. The baby is likely to be compromised after a total spinal from maternal hypoxia and hypotension even without maternal cardiac arrest. Urgent delivery may be necessary.

Once the woman has been resuscitated, anesthetic agents (especially intravenous drugs if the woman is not in the operating room) will be needed to keep her asleep. Owing to the paralyzing effect of the block, she may be conscious but unable to move or communicate. She should be verbally reassured. Paralysis, analgesia, and the inability to talk may last for less than 1 hour but it may take several hours for the block to wear off. It is possible to manage this situation in the operating room or the post-anesthesia care unit, or the woman may require transfer to the intensive care unit.

Local anesthetic toxicity

Introduction

Local anesthetics are widely used in obstetrics.[2] As with all interventions, local anesthetics are not without risk and have been associated with deaths. One of the six deaths attributable to anesthesia reported in the Confidential Enquiry into Maternal Deaths 2003–05 was the result of a drug administration error:[1]

> "A woman of slight build had a low-dose infusion epidural during labor and was delivered by forceps. She had some bleeding and intravenous fluid and oxytocin infusions were started. Shortly after, she had a grand mal convulsion followed by ventricular fibrillation from which she could not be resuscitated. She had received 150 ml of a 500 ml bag of 0.1% bupivacaine in saline intravenously in error."

This was a system error, as a bag of epidural bupivacaine should never have been confused with a bag of intravenous fluid. Nevertheless, it demonstrates the danger of local anesthetics if unintentionally intravenously administered.

The National Reporting and Learning Service of the National Patient Safety Agency (NPSA) published several safety alerts advising on strategies to avoid such errors. Initial recommendations focused on clear labeling and the use of equipment specifically designed for epidural injections and infusions.[12] Further recommendations include all spinal (intrathecal) injections be performed using syringes, needles, and other devices with connectors that would not also connect with intravenous equipment.[13] This has been extended to all epidural and regional anesthesia infusions and bolus doses.[14]

Signs and symptoms of local anesthetic toxicity

Local anesthetic toxicity can present in many different ways, making recognition difficult. It is important to remember that after epidural injection of a bolus dose of local anesthetic, toxicity may occur immediately (from unrecognized intravascular injection) or virtually at any point over the next hour from absorption and circulation of a large dose of local anesthetic. More recently, the growing use of epidural infusions has led to a rising incidence of local anesthetic toxicity during labor (see example above). The features to look for are shown in Table 4.1.

Remember: the first sign may be cardiac arrest.

Table 4.1 Signs and symptoms of toxicity

Warning signs	■ Tingling (mouth/tongue)	
	■ Metallic taste in the mouth	
	■ Ringing in the ears	
	■ Lightheadedness	
	■ Agitation ("just not right")	
	■ Tremor	
Severe toxicity	**Neurological**	**Cardiovascular**
	■ Severe agitation	■ Bradycardia
	■ Loss of consciousness	■ Heart block
	■ Convulsions	■ Ventricular tachyarrythmias
		■ Asystole/cardiac arrest

Management

All healthcare professionals caring for women with epidurals should be familiar with the management of severe local anesthetic toxicity,[15] an outline of which is illustrated in Table 4.2. The lipid emulsion regimen is shown in Figure 4.5.

Specific treatment for local anesthetic toxicity

Local anesthetic toxicity has successfully been treated with an intravenous infusion of lipid emulsion, commercially known as Intralipid® (Baxter Healthcare Corporation, Deerfield, IL, USA). Intralipid® has also been reported to improve survival from local-anesthetic-induced cardiac arrest[16,17] and in the treatment of life-threatening toxicity without cardiac arrest.[18] It does not replace the need for CPR, which should continue throughout treatment with lipid emulsion until the return of spontaneous circulation. It should be noted that cardiac arrest secondary to local anesthetic toxicity can be refractory to treatment, perhaps requiring rebolus and titration of Intralipid® infusion. Recovery may take over 1 hour. Thus the effort of a large number of people is required to ensure that good quality CPR is maintained throughout.

> **Remember: know where lipid emulsion is kept in your department.**

Severe local anesthetic toxicity is a rare but very serious complication of local anesthetic use. Posters should be used to remind staff of the salient points and, most importantly, where to find treatment guidelines and lipid emulsion should they ever be faced with this emergency.

Follow-up

The management of local-anesthetic-induced cardiac arrest is very demanding. If successful, transfer to a critical care area will need to be arranged until full recovery is achieved.

Each case should be reported. The lessons learned can potentially prevent other cases from happening and improve our knowledge and treatment of the condition. All cases where lipid emulsion has been given should be reported to the international registry at www.lipidregistry.org.

Table 4.2 Management of severe local anesthetic toxicity

Immediate management	■ Stop injecting local anesthetic	
	■ Call for help	
	■ Maintain airway; intubate if necessary	
	■ Give 100% oxygen and ensure adequate ventilation	
	■ Confirm/establish IV access	
	■ Control seizures	
	■ Assess cardiovascular status throughout	
Treatment	**In cardiac arrest**	**Without cardiac arrest**

	■ Commence advanced life support using standard algorithm with woman supine and uterus manually displaced to the left	■ Use conventional therapies to treat:
		  ☐ Hypotension
		  ☐ Bradycardia
		  ☐ Tachyarrythmias

	■ Treat arrhythmias using standard protocols	■ Consider intravenous lipid emulsion
	■ Give intravenous lipid emulsion (follow regimen shown in Figure 4.5)	■ Keep woman in left-lateral tilt
	■ Continue CPR throughout treatment with lipid emulsion	
	■ Recovery may take longer than 1 hour	
Special points	■ Propofol is not a suitable substitute for lipid emulsion	
	■ Arrhythmias may be very refractory to treatment	
	■ Lidocaine should not be used as an anti-arrhythmic in this setting	

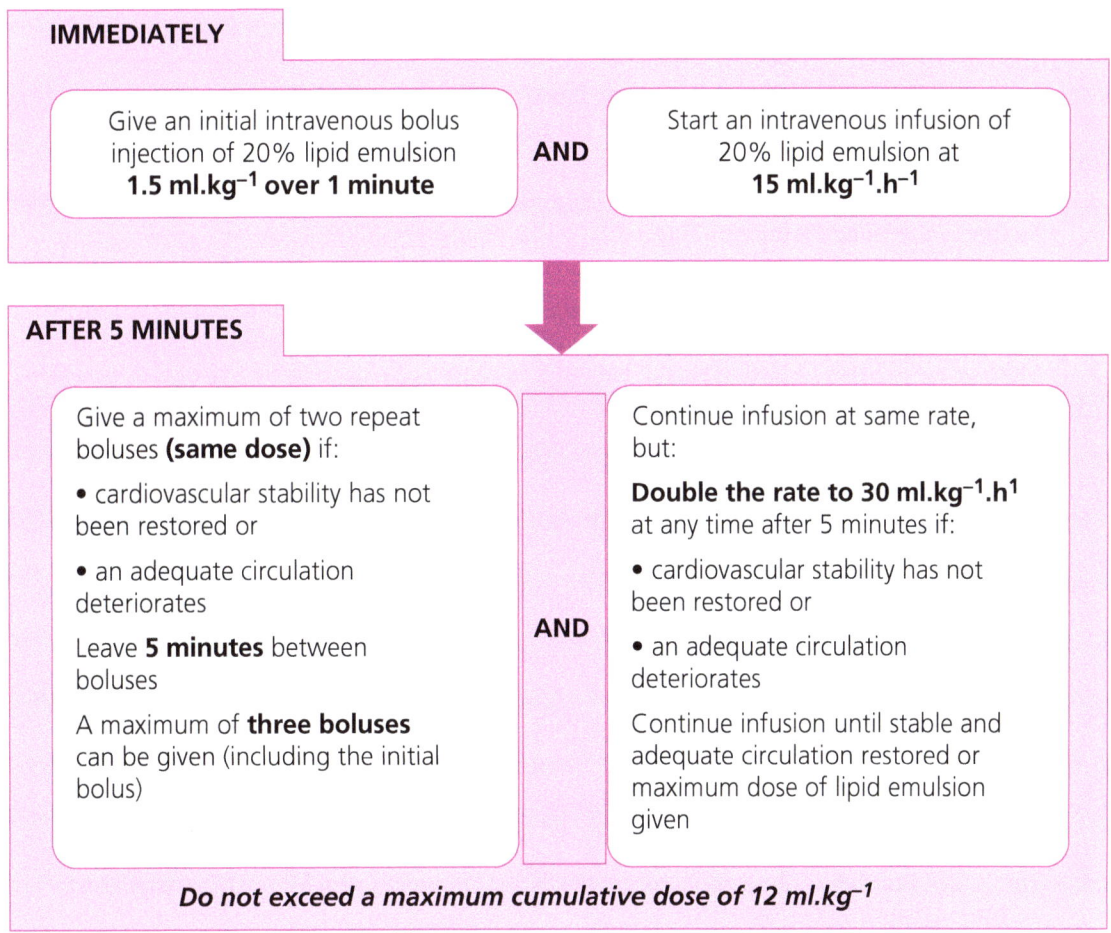

An approximate dose regimen for a 70 kg woman would be as follows:

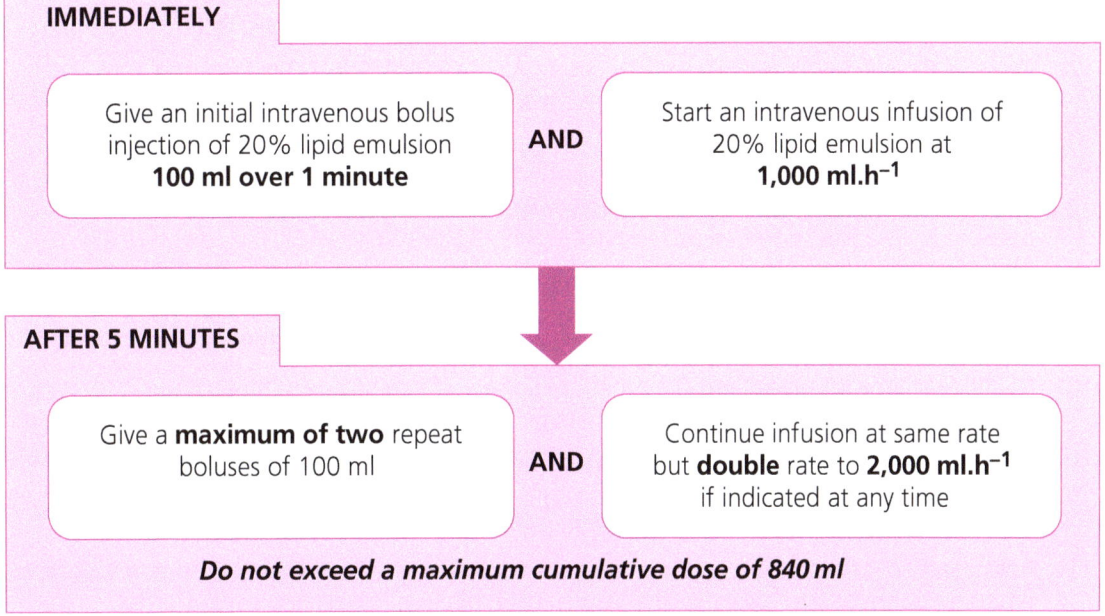

Figure 4.5 Intravenous lipid emulsion regimen (©Association of Anaesthetists of Great Britain & Ireland 2010, reproduced with permission)

References

1. Creanga AA, Berg CJ, Syverson C, Seed K, Bruce FC, Callaghan WM. Pregnancy-related mortality in the United States, 2006–2010. *Obstet Gynecol* 2015; 125: 5-12.

2. Centre for Maternal and Child Enquiries. Saving Mothers' Lives: reviewing maternal deaths to make motherhood safer: 2006–08. The Eighth Report on Confidential Enquiries into Maternal Deaths in the United Kingdom. *BJOG* 2011; 118 (Suppl 1): 1–203.

3. Knight M, Kenyon S, Brocklehurst P, Neilson J, Shakespeare J, Kurinczuk JJ (eds) on behalf of MBRRACE-UK. *Saving Lives, Improving Mothers' Care: Lessons Learned to Inform Future Maternity Care from the UK and Ireland Confidential Enquiries into Maternal Deaths and Morbidity 2009–12*. Oxford: National Perinatal Epidemiology Unit, University of Oxford; 2014.

4. Hospital Episode Statistics. *NHS Maternity Statistics, 2009–2010*. London: The Health and Social Care Information Centre; 2010 [www.hesonline.nhs.uk/Ease/servlet/ContentServer?siteID=1937&categoryID=1804].

5. McGlennan A, Mustafa A. General anaesthesia for Caesarean section. *Contin Educ Anaesth Crit Care Pain* 2009; 9: 148–51.

6. Centre for Maternal and Child Enquiries, Royal College of Obstetricians and Gynaecologists. *CMACE/RCOG Joint Guideline. Management of Women with Obesity in Pregnancy*. London: CMACE/RCOG; 2010 [www.rcog.org.uk/womens-health/clinical-guidance/management-women-obesity-pregnancy].

7. Collins JS, Lemmens HJ, Brodsky JB, Brock-Utne JG, Levitan RM. Laryngoscopy and morbid obesity: a comparison of the "sniff" and "ramped" positions. *Obes Surg* 2004; 14: 1171–5.

8. Mhyre JM, Healy D. The unanticipated difficult intubation in obstetrics. *Anesth Analg* 2011; 112: 648–52.

9. Yentis SM, Dob DP. High regional block: the failed intubation of the new millennium? *Int J Obstet Anaesth* 2001; 10: 159–61.

10. Allman K, McIndoe A, Wilson I (eds) *Emergencies in Anaesthesia, 2nd edn*. Oxford: Oxford University Press; 2009.

11. Jenkins JG. Some immediate serious complications of obstetric epidural analgesia and anaesthesia: a prospective study of 145,550 epidurals. *Int J Obstet Anest* 2005; 14: 37–42.

12. National Patient Safety Agency. *Patient Safety Alert NPSA/2007/21: Epidural Injections and Infusions*. London: NPSA; 2007 [www.nrls.npsa.nhs.uk/resources/?entryid45=59807 &q=0%C2%AC2007%2f21%C2%AC].

13. National Patient Safety Agency. *Patient Safety Alert NPSA/2009/PSA004B: Safer Spinal (Intrathecal), Epidural and Regional Devices – Part B*. London: NPSA; 2009 [www.nrls.npsa.nhs.uk/resources/?entryid45=94529&q=0%C2%ACsafer+spinal%C2%AC].

14. National Patient Safety Agency. *Patient Safety Alert NPSA/2009/PSA004A: Safer Spinal (Intrathecal), Epidural and Regional Devices – Part A (Update)*. London: NPSA; 2011 [www.nrls.npsa.nhs.uk/resources/?entryid45=94529&q=0%C2%ACsafer+spinal%C2%AC].

15. Neal JM, Mulroy MF, Weinberg GL. American Society of Regional Anesthesia and Pain Medicine checklist for managing local anesthetic systemic toxicity: 2012 version. *Reg Anesth Pain Med* 2012; 37: 16–8.

16. Weinberg G, Ripper R, Feinstein DL, Hoffman W. Lipid emulsion infusion rescues dogs from bupivacaine-induced cardiac toxicity. *Reg Anaesth Pain Med* 2003; 28: 198–202.

17. Rosenblatt MA, Abel M, Fischer GW, Itzkovich CJ, Eisenkraft JB. Successful use of a 20% lipid emulsion to resuscitate a patient after a presumed bupivacaine-related cardiac arrest. *Anesthesiology* 2006; 105: 217–18.

18. Foxall G, McCahon R, Lamb J, Hardman JG, Bedforth NM. Levobupivacaine-induced seizures and cardiovascular collapse treated with Intralipid. *Anaesthesia* 2007; 62: 516–18.

Module 5
Fetal monitoring in labor

Problems identified from case discussions

■ Not documenting the fetal heart simultaneously using either an ultrasound or a Pinard stethoscope when starting EFM to confirm the signal is the fetal heart rate.

■ Not documenting a systematic assessment of the EFM pattern at least hourly.

■ Not involving experienced practitioners to assist decision-making when the EFM pattern is difficult to interpret.

- Not documenting and signing all relevant interventions and EFM pattern interpretations on the appropriate section of the tracing in addition to the labor record.

- Not making an appropriate plan for timely review of the EFM tracing.

- Not continuing EFM until birth, particularly if the mother is transferred out of the labor room, e.g., if delivery occurs in the OR.

Introduction

Fetal heart rate measurement has been a key assessment of fetal health during labor for over 200 years: a poem written by Phillipe Le Goust in 1650 refers to hearing the fetal heart "beating like the clapper of a mill...". The Pinard stethoscope was introduced in 1876 for intermittent auscultation, and in 1893 Von Winkel established criteria for determining potential "fetal distress," some of which are still used today: fetal tachycardia over 160 beats/minute (bpm), fetal bradycardia less than 100 bpm and gross alteration of fetal movements.[1]

Electronic fetal heart rate monitoring was introduced in 1958. At that time, it was not uncommon for babies to die in labor with apparently few warning signs. Thus the original goal of EFM was to prevent intrapartum fetal deaths. It was later assumed that EFM would also lead to earlier detection of hypoxia, allowing a more timely intervention to reduce cerebral palsy (CP) rates. It is important to understand that during that time period, it was assumed most cases of CP were caused by intrapartum fetal hypoxia. We now know only about 10% of CP cases are related to intrapartum events, and occult inflammation is increasingly implicated as a cause of CP, independent of labor.[2,3]

Routine intrapartum EFM rapidly entered mainstream care despite little proof of efficacy. Meta-analysis of randomized controlled trials of EFM compared with intermittent auscultation demonstrated no difference in perinatal outcome between the two, although EFM was associated with an increased risk of operative delivery, particularly cesarean section. Though rarely employed in North America, operative intervention rates are reduced when fetal blood sampling is used as an adjunct to EFM.[4,5]

It has been suggested that the lack of improvement in perinatal outcome despite the use of EFM can be attributed to the insufficient sample size of most randomized trials, as very large studies (35,000 women) are required to determine the efficacy of EFM. The largest intrapartum fetal monitoring trial, the Dublin trial, noted a reduction in neonatal seizures in the EFM arm but no difference in long-term outcome.[6] The trial was not powered to detect differences in rates of CP.

It is often overlooked that most randomized trials of EFM and intermittent auscultation conclude neither method is particularly reliable, and that there are important "human" factors affecting outcome. Poor skill of healthcare personnel interpreting EFM patterns and the resulting failure to take appropriate action remain central problems and may contribute to the failure of EFM to reduce perinatal mortality. Murphy et al. observed pattern abnormalities were missed by healthcare providers in both the EFM and intermittent auscultation groups in 64 cases of significant birth asphyxia.[7] Such problems are recurring themes in both the US Joint Commission on Accreditation of Healthcare (JACHO) and the UK Confidential Enquiry into Stillbirths and Deaths in Infancy (CESDI) reports.[8, 9, 10] Grant succinctly noted that "for monitoring to be effective, it must be performed correctly, its results must then be interpreted satisfactorily, and this interpretation must provoke an appropriate response."[4]

One large perinatal review concluded that 70% of intrapartum deaths had avoidable factors, notably a lack of understanding of EFM pattern interpretation.[11] Similar experiences by others have led to the widespread recommendation that regular training and updates in EFM pattern interpretation be implemented.[11] In 2008, the Eunice Kennedy Shriver National Institute of Child Health and Human Development (NICHD), the American College of Obstetricians and Gynecologists (ACOG), and the Society for Maternal-Fetal Medicine (SMFM) jointly sponsored a two-day workshop to revisit and standardize nomenclature, interpretation, and provide research recommendations for intrapartum EFM. In an attempt to simplify the process of interpretation and thus improve consistency, the panel proposed a three-tiered categorization: the good, the bad, and the ugly – better known as Category I, II, and III.[12] Though this consensus approach has become the standard in the United States, it remains unclear whether it achieves the desired goal of interpretation consistency, or whether its application results in improved clinical outcomes.

Risk management and training

Both intrapartum death and the birth of a baby with severe brain damage are tragedies for families and society. The evidence linking brain injury to intrapartum care is inconsistent but remains a major trigger for litigation.[13,14] The basis of many claims includes:

- intermittent auscultation was too infrequent
- failure to recognize an abnormal EFM pattern

■ failure to act on an abnormal EFM pattern

■ failure to call medical staff soon enough or often enough.[15]

A Swedish study reviewed the outcomes of infants delivered after 33 weeks between 2004 and 2006 and found evidence of substandard care during labor in two-thirds of infants with a five-minute Apgar score below 7. The main reasons for the substandard care judgment were misinterpretation of the EFM pattern, not acting on an abnormal pattern in a timely fashion, and imprudent use of oxytocin.[16] Substandard care is unlikely to be defensible if a poor outcome results, and litigation is expensive; individual claims exceed $20 million (US). Adequate interpretation and documentation of the EFM is crucial to quality improvement and the reduction of medico-legal risk. While similar granular data is unavailable in the United States, claims for damaged babies in the UK account for more than half of the annual total National Health Service (NHS) litigation bill.[17]

All practitioners providing intrapartum care should have the knowledge and skills to interpret EFM tracings and act appropriately, with the aim of providing high-quality, defensible care. Each individual obstetric unit should provide regular fetal heart rate monitoring training for all relevant staff in line with national recommendations.[18]

Draycott et al. demonstrated mandatory skills training in EFM tracing interpretation and obstetric emergencies improved neonatal outcomes in one UK maternity unit, and the Northern California Kaiser Permanente Perinatal Patient Safety Program described an improved safety climate after training.[19,20] Important, but typically lacking in programs, training should cover not only EFM interpretation, but also the skills required to communicate the interpretation and the actions of the team responding to an emergency. This suggests improving outcomes in labor when EFM is used is probably dependent on more than just EFM interpretation training alone. A systematic review by Pehrson et al. concluded that training can improve EFM interpretation competence and clinical practice, but further research is needed to evaluate the type and content of training that is most effective.[21]

Physiology and pathophysiology

The healthy fetus is able to cope with the stresses of labor and adapts appropriately to meet the challenge. Current evidence supports the use of intermittent auscultation for "low-risk" mothers.

Fetal oxygen supply

In comparison with adults, the fetal partial pressure of oxygen is relatively low; however, the fetus has a remarkable margin of safety. A high concentration of fetal hemoglobin and its greater affinity for absorbing oxygen means that oxygen saturation is high. The cardiac output of the fetus is also efficient. As a result, the fetal oxygen supply is usually greater than requirements.

Fetal gas exchange is impaired during uterine contractions, which means oxygen levels fall and carbon dioxide (CO_2) levels increase. Between contractions, the oxygen supply is restored and the accumulated CO_2 is excreted. Conditions that impair gas exchange within the placenta, such as hypercontractility, umbilical cord occlusion, maternal hypotension, or placental abruption, all acutely cause CO_2 retention, which lowers the pH of the fetal blood (respiratory acidosis). This should resolve when placental perfusion is restored (approximately 2 minutes for every minute the fetal heart rate (FHR) is below 90 bpm in a term fetus). However, if gas exchange continues to be impeded, the fetus must rely on other important defense mechanisms:

- **Hormonal response**
  A reduction in fetal oxygen is detected by chemoreceptors in the fetal aorta. This activates a hormonal response with an increase in catecholamines, vasopressin, adenine, and adenosine levels. Catecholamine levels in the asphyxiated neonate can exceed those of patients with pheochromocytoma.[22]

- **Preferential redistribution of blood flow**
  Over time, there is decreased blood flow to non-"essential" organs such as the liver, spleen, intestine, kidneys, and skin. Blood supply to "priority" organs – brain, heart, and adrenal glands – increases through a combination of vasodilation and increased fetal cardiac output. Myocardial blood flow can increase up to 500% in response to hypoxia. Oxygen requirements for the brain are not as great and fetal behavior can adapt to reduce energy requirements.

- **Glycogenolysis**
  When the oxygen supply is no longer sufficient to meet the fetal energy requirements, the release of epinephrine activates glycogenolysis and increases the fetal cardiac rate. Glucose is released from glycogen stores and metabolized anaerobically (without oxygen) to maintain energy requirements.

Stores of glycogen in the heart, muscle, and liver are broken down to provide energy. Lactic acid, a by-product of anaerobic metabolism, is initially buffered (neutralized) but will eventually cause the pH of the blood to fall further

Box 5.1 Factors that influence fetal oxygenation		
Mother	**Uterus/placenta**	**Fetus**
Anemia	Abruption	Anemia
Analgesia/anesthesia	Umbilical cord prolapse	Fetal bleeding
Dehydration	Impaired placental function	Infection
Hypertension	Uterine hypercontractility	Growth restriction
Hypotension		
Pyrexia		

(metabolic acidosis). As the fetus continues to use glycogen stores, the acidosis becomes predominantly metabolic in origin and the pH decreases even further.

Conditions and events that affect the mother (e.g., pre-eclampsia, diabetes, antepartum hemorrhage) and/or placental function (e.g., too frequent or prolonged uterine contractions, abruption) and/or fetal defense mechanisms (chronic hypoxemia [IUGR], infection and stress) may render the fetus less able to adapt and more vulnerable to either chronic or acute hypoxia (Box 5.1).

Compensatory responses and adaptation to hypoxia can protect the fetus for only a finite amount of time. When the defense mechanisms are blunted, depleted, or overwhelmed, the risk of perinatal asphyxia (hypoxia, acidosis, and tissue damage) is increased.

Standards for intermittent auscultation during labor

Though an uncommon choice in much of North America, intermittent auscultation may be used to monitor fetal wellbeing when the mother is healthy and has an uncomplicated pregnancy with either a Doppler ultrasound or a Pinard stethoscope.[15]

In active labor:

- 1st stage: intermittent auscultation at least every 15 minutes after a contraction and for a minimum of 60 seconds. Count the fetal heart rate over a full minute and record the rate on the labor record.[23]

- 2nd stage: intermittent auscultation every 5 minutes after a contraction and for a minimum of a full minute.

- Any intrapartum event that may affect the fetal heart rate should be noted contemporaneously in the nursing notes, signed, and timed.

- If a fetal heart rate abnormality is suspected, the maternal pulse should be palpated simultaneously with the fetal heart to differentiate between the two heart rates.

Continuous EFM is recommended when:

- the baseline is below 110 bpm or greater than 160 bpm on intermittent auscultation
- any decelerations are suspected after a contraction
- any intrapartum risk factors develop (Figure 5.1).

The current evidence does not support the use of an admission FHR strip as a screening tool in low-risk pregnancies.[15]

Technical considerations for EFM in labor

In most North American hospitals, a pulse oximeter is placed on each laboring woman, and the transcutaneous oxygen saturation and maternal pulse printed contemporaneously on the EFM tracing. If continuous maternal pulse oximetry is not being used, it is best to auscultate the fetal heart using a Pinard stethoscope (or visualize it using ultrasound) rather than a Doppler before starting EFM since it is possible to generate a signal from a large, pulsating maternal vessel, which can be misinterpreted as the fetal heart rate. Furthermore, the ultrasound software may falsely double the maternal pulse rate if there is sufficient separation between valve movements, generating a rate that would be within normal for the fetus. Absent use of a pulse oximeter, the maternal pulse should also be palpated regularly with any form of fetal heart rate monitoring to differentiate between maternal and fetal heart rates. There have been occasional reports of unexpected macerated stillbirths with apparently normal intrapartum EFM patterns, even with direct fetal scalp electrode application.[24,25]

All members of staff should be aware of the technical limitations of EFM and read the manufacturer's instructions for each particular monitor.

Standards for electronic fetal monitoring

While the use of EFM has become the de facto standard in many North American hospitals, its ubiquitous use contributes to unnecessary operative intervention. It is important to document the accuracy of the written record, especially if the EFM tracing is not going to be stored in digital format.

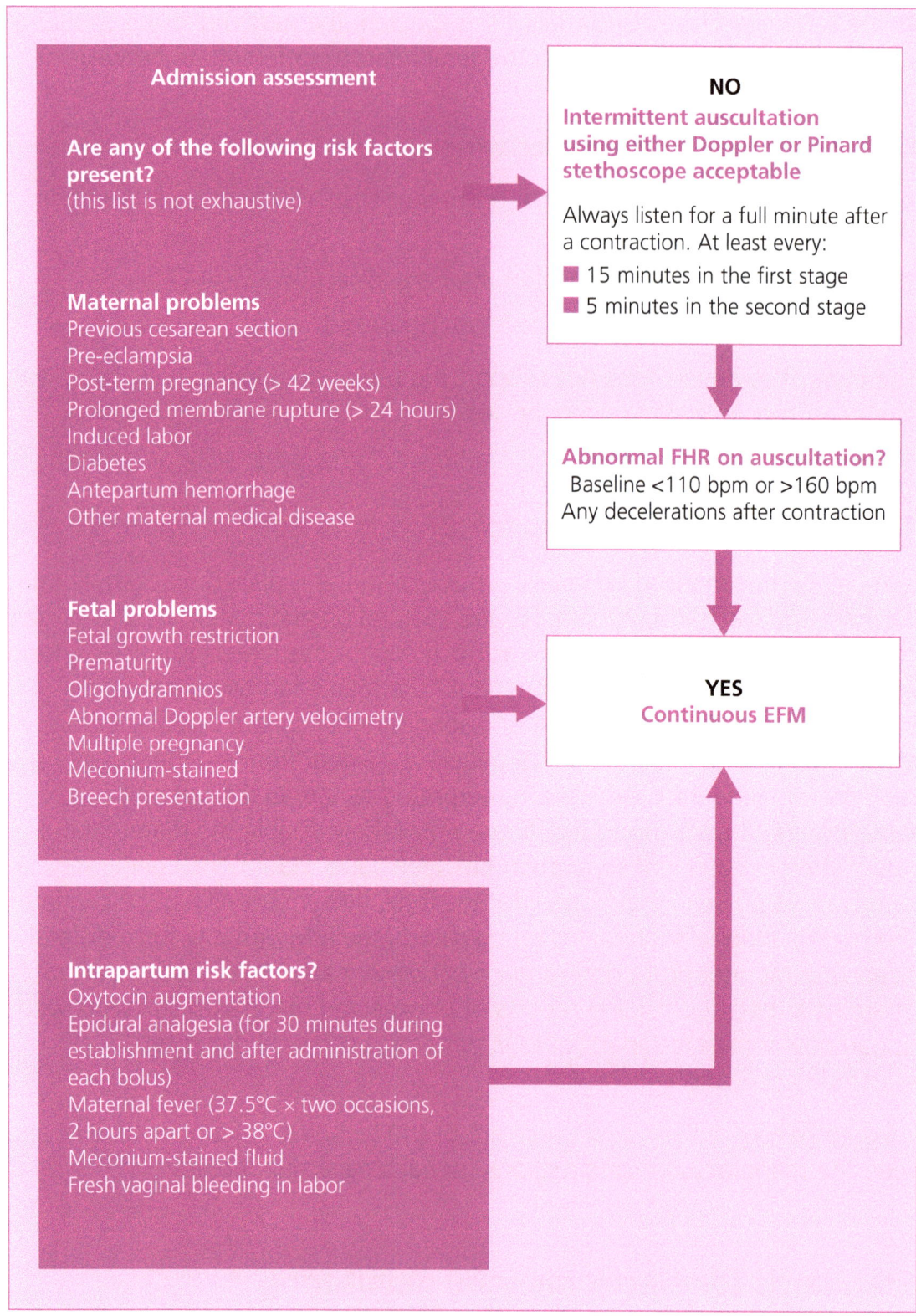

Figure 5.1 Admission assessment with fetal monitoring in labor

EFM check list (attach to start the first part of the tracing)	
Reason for EFM:	
Date:	Date set correctly on monitor? (check)
Time:	Time set correctly on monitor? (check)
Name:	
Hospital number:	Gestation:
	Maternal pulse (rate):
(or attach addressograph)	FH auscultated prior to EFM if no pulse oximeter (rate):
Attach to end of the EFM tracing	
Mode of delivery:	Date of birth:
Signature:	Time of birth:

Figure 5.2 Example of start and end stickers to attach to the EFM tracing if not stored digitally

- The date and time clocks on the machine should be correct and paper speed set to 3 cm/minute in the United States and 1 cm/minute in Canada (Figure 5.2).
- The EFM paper should be labeled with the mother's name and hospital number and dated (Figure 5.2).
- Any intrapartum event that may affect the fetal heart rate should be noted contemporaneously on the paper or electronic strip, signed, and dated (such as vaginal examinations, fetal blood sampling, epidural insertion, and bolus doses).
- If external EFM monitoring is not of sufficient quality for interpretation, then a fetal scalp electrode should be applied if possible.
- Following delivery, the caregiver should sign, date, time, and list mode of delivery on the EFM tracing (Figure 5.2).
- The EFM trace should be stored securely.

Features of the intrapartum EFM tracing and terminology

Most clinicians have no difficulty recognizing the features of a normal intrapartum EFM tracing, as shown in Figures 5.3a–c. However, it is important

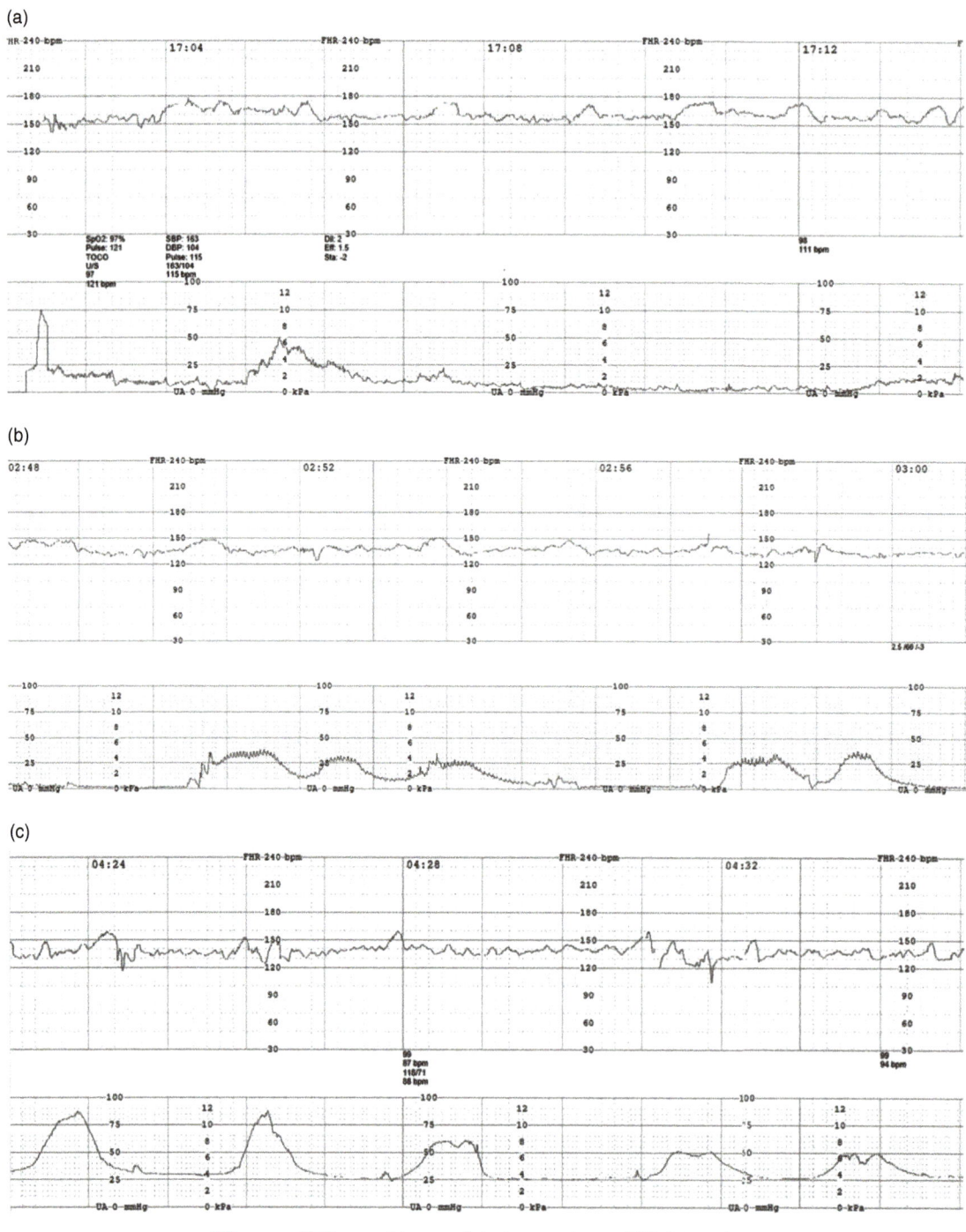

Figure 5.3a–c Normal intrapartum EFM tracing

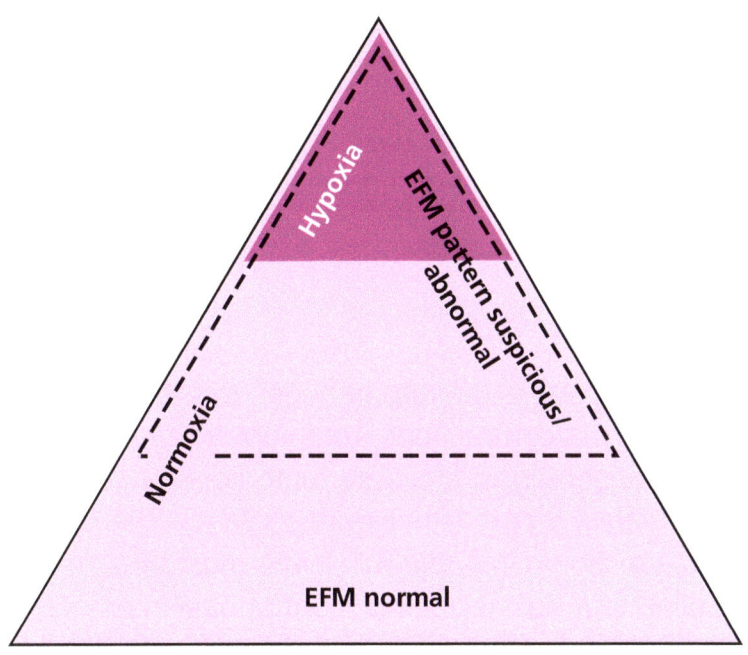

Figure 5.4 Relationship between EFM tracing and fetal oxygenation

to remember that a suspicious pattern does not necessarily mean the fetus is hypoxic (insufficient oxygen to meet metabolic requirements). In fact, this is often not the case, as illustrated in Figure 5.4. The sensitivity of EFM pattern recognition for hypoxia is high; you can conclude a fetus is not significantly hypoxic when the EFM pattern is normal. However, the specificity of interpretation is low if the pattern is abnormal – only about 50% of fetuses will show some degree of hypoxia. It remains useful to perform a fetal scalp pH whenever the interpretation of the pattern is unclear if you have been so trained.

There is no reliable way to determine fetal oxygen reserve. The growth-restricted fetus may have a blunted response due to adaptation to chronic stress and inadequate glycogen stores, and an acute event may quickly overwhelm the defense mechanisms of even a healthy baby. Such fetuses often have abnormal Doppler waveforms in multiple fetal organs. The EFM pattern must always be interpreted in the context of the antepartum and intrapartum clinical history and events.

It is essential that communications between all healthcare providers describe the features of the intrapartum EFM tracing using consistent terminology, the level of concern, and the urgency of the situation.

There are four main features that should be systematically examined whenever interpreting the tracing:

- baseline rate
- baseline variability

■ accelerations
■ decelerations.

These features, in conjunction with the contraction pattern and the clinical circumstances, should all be considered when deciding whether to take any action.

Baseline fetal heart rate

The baseline fetal heart rate is the rate between events that have the potential to alter that rate, such as contractions, fetal movements, and fetal heart rate accelerations and decelerations. It is determined over a 10-minute period and expressed to the nearest 5 bpm (see Figures 5.3a–c). The ranges and descriptive terms are shown in Table 5.1.There must be at least 2 minutes of identifiable baseline (but not necessarily contiguous) in any 10-minute window, or the baseline for that period is indeterminate. In that instance, it may be necessary to refer to the previous 10-minute window for determination of the baseline.

Baseline variability

Baseline variability consists of minor fluctuations in the baseline fetal heart rate normally occurring at three to five cycles/minute (see Figures 5.3a–c). The presence of normal variability is one of the most important findings. The current standard in the United States is to describe variability in terms of the

Table 5.1 Baseline ranges

Level	Rate (beats/minute)
Reassuring	
Normal baseline	110–160
Not reassuring	
Moderate bradycardia	100–109
Moderate tachycardia[a]	161–180
Abnormal	
Abnormal bradycardia	<100
Abnormal tachycardia	>180

[a] A tachycardia of 161–180 beats/minute, where accelerations are present and no other adverse features appear, should NOT be regarded as suspicious. However, an increase in the baseline rate, even within the normal range, with other non-reassuring or abnormal features should increase concern.[14]

height of those cycles above baseline – **absent**: amplitude range undetectable; **minimal**: amplitude range > undetectable and ≤5 bpm; **moderate**: amplitude range 6–25 bpm; and **marked**: amplitude range >25 bpm.

Accelerations

Accelerations are an abrupt, transient increase in the fetal heart rate variably defined according to gestational age. The tracing is considered to be **reactive** when there are at least two accelerations that exceed 15 bpm above baseline for at least 15 seconds at gestational age of 32 weeks or greater, or if less than 32 weeks, 10 bpm above baseline for at least 10 seconds (Figures 5.3a–c). Reactivity does not exclude mild to moderate fetal hypoxia, but does exclude significant fetal acidemia and when employed for antenatal monitoring suggests the fetus is unlikely to die within seven days if the intrauterine environment is stable. For that reason, a reactive tracing is reassuring. The absence of accelerations with an otherwise normal EFM pattern is also considered inconsistent with significant fetal acidosis; repeated accelerations associated with reduced variability is also regarded as reassuring.[15]

Decelerations

Decelerations are a transient slowing of the fetal heart rate below the baseline level; some suggest they should be at least for 15 seconds. There are fundamentally two basic types of waveforms – uniform (in shape, timing, occurrence, and the magnitude of the deceleration reflects the magnitude of the contraction) and non-uniform. The importance of deceleration depth likely reflects the underlying mechanism.

Variable decelerations:	These are the most common decelerations seen during labor. A non-uniform, periodic slowing of the fetal heart rate, with rapid onset and recovery. Time relationships with contraction cycle are variable and the decelerations can occur in isolation. They may resemble other types of decelerations in terms of their timing and shape, but they do not do so with uniformity. They are caused by umbilical cord compression and can be typical or atypical in appearance (Figure 5.5a–c).
	Typical variable decelerations (Figure 5.5a) are an autonomic response to cord compression and demonstrate the fetus has the capacity to cope with the stress of labor. Think of them as analogous to breath

holding. The longer and more frequently the fetus holds its breath, the higher the CO_2 climbs. The fetus will clear the CO_2 if there is adequate time between declerations. Over time, the fetus may accumulate lactate at a rate greater than which occurs normally in labor.

The level of scrutiny should be increased if the decelerations are frequent (more than 50% of contractions for more than 90 minutes*) and/or there is any suspected fetal compromise such as growth restriction.[16] Atypical variable decelerations may subsequently develop, indicating that the fetus is beginning to lose the capacity to cope.

Atypical variable decelerations are variable decelerations with any of the following components (Figures 5.5b,c):

- loss of the primary or secondary rise in baseline rate (loss of the shoulder)
- slow return to the fetal heart rate baseline after the contraction ends
- prolonged secondary rise in baseline rate (exaggerated shoulder)
- a biphasic deceleration
- continuation of baseline rate at lower level.

Atypical variable decelerations occurring with more than half the contractions for more than 30 minutes should be considered high risk and subject to further action.[15]

* It may be unwise to wait 90 minutes (typical variable) or 30 minutes (atypical variable) to notify the obstetrician if the FHR tracing shows typical or atypical variable decelerations from the outset of EFM.

Late decelerations: These are uniform decelerations with their onset well after the onset of the contraction and their nadir after the peak of the contraction (typically after the end of the contraction). Late decelerations are caused by hypoxia (not acidemia), and if associated with diminished variability and absent accelerations for more than 30 minutes,** are considered indicative of a degree of fetal hypoxia in need of further action (Figures 5.6 a,b).[15]

** It may not be wise to wait 30 minutes to notify the obstetrician if the FHR tracing shows late decelerations from the start of the tracing.

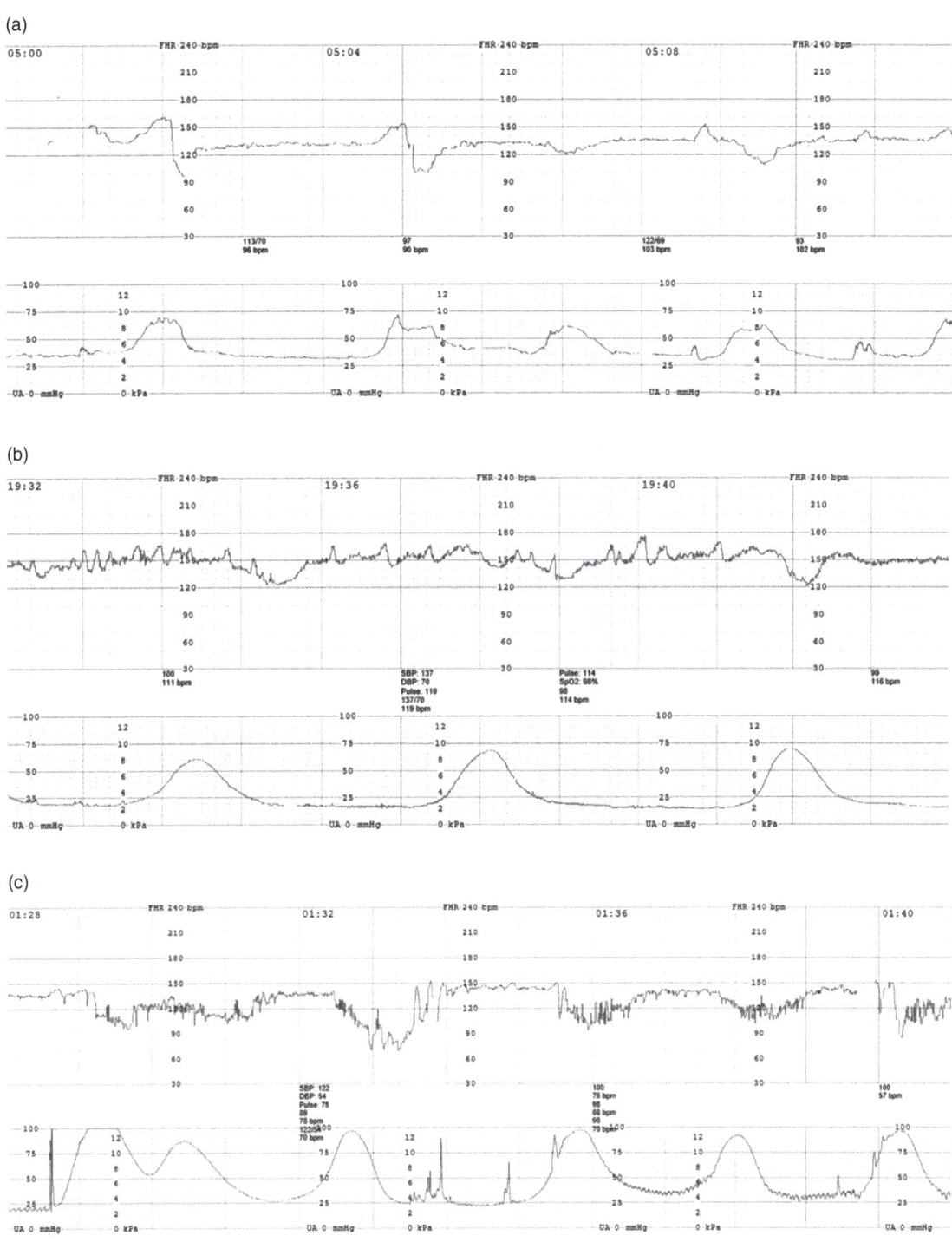

Figure 5.5 (a) Typical variable decelerations; **(b, c)** atypical variable decelerations (3 cm/min)

Early decelerations: Another uniform decleration, but in contrast to the late deceleration, it begins early in the contraction and returns to baseline by the end of the contraction (Figure 5.7). The lowest point of the deceleration typically coincides with the contraction peak. Early decelerations are usually associated with head compression and thus tend to occur late in the 1st stage or during the 2nd stage of labor. True early decelerations are uncommon (often confused with variable decelerations) and benign; they are not associated with fetal hypoxia.

(a)

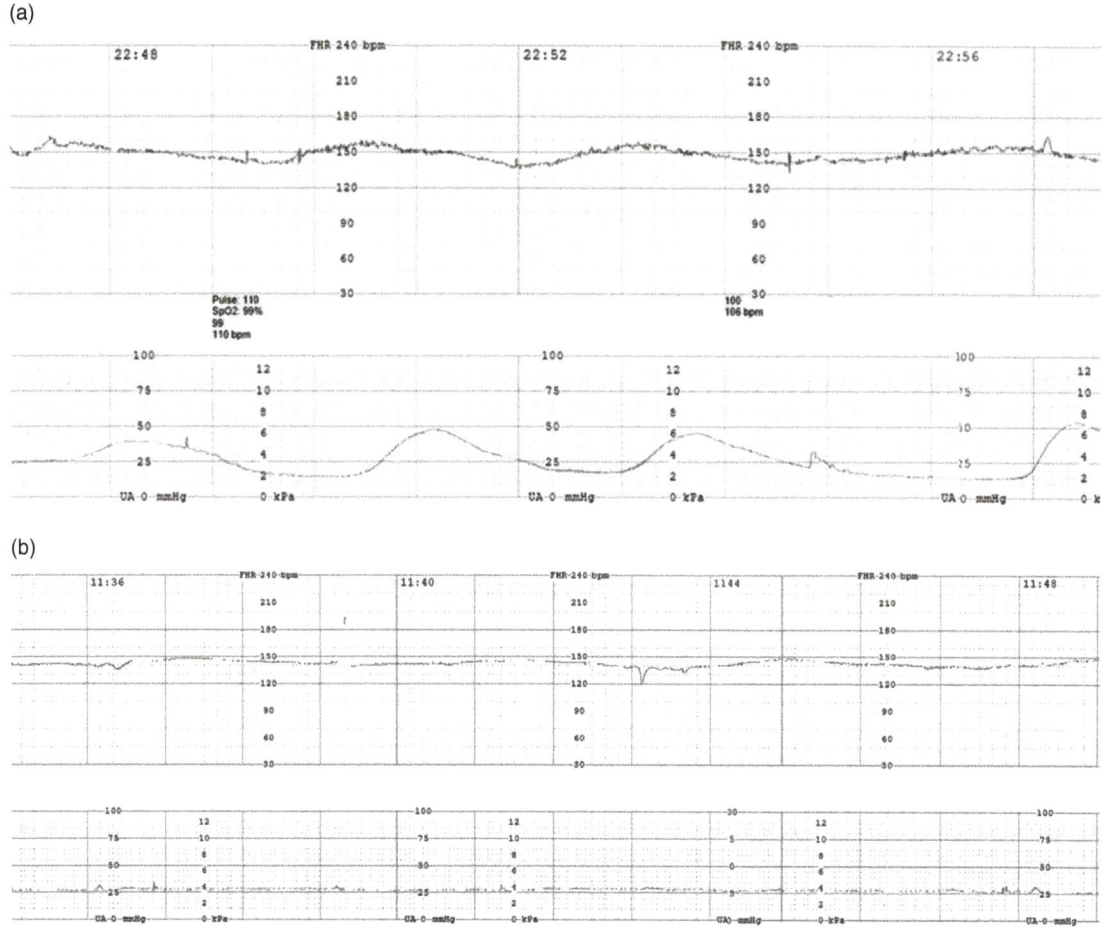

(b)

Figures 5.6 a,b Late decelerations (3 cm/min)

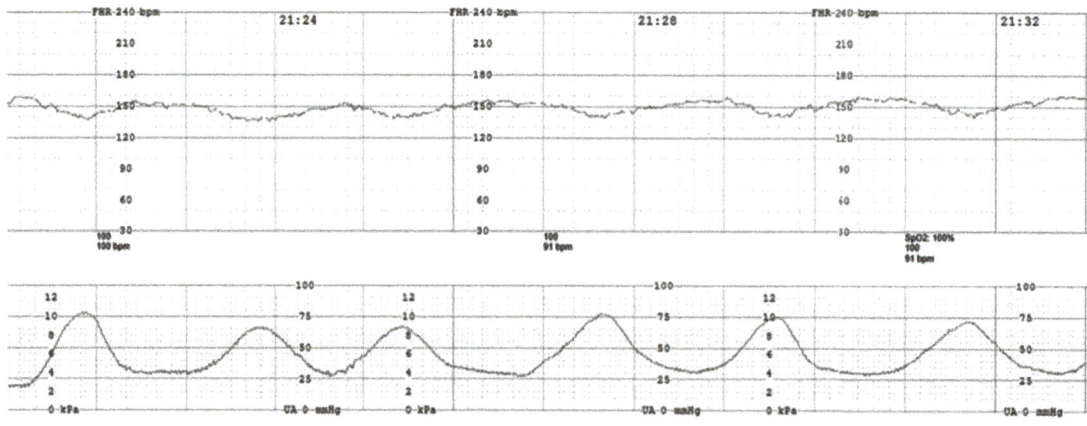

Figure 5.7 Early decelerations (3 cm/min)

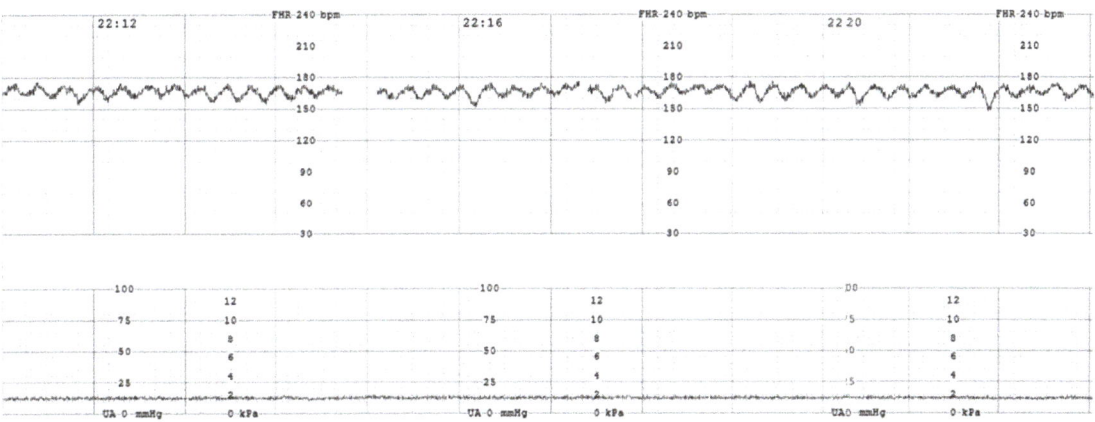

Figure 5.8 Sinusoidal pattern (3 cm/min)

Prolonged deceleration: An abrupt decline in the fetal heart rate below baseline that lasts more than 2 but less than 10 minutes. If the rate is lower than 90 bpm and lasts more than 3 minutes, plans should be made to expedite delivery using the most appropriate method. The fetal pH declines by about 0.03 units per minute under 90 bpm while the $_pCO_2$ increases by about 4 mmHg per minute. An emergency should be declared and the patient immediately transferred to the OR. If the fetal heart has recovered to above 90 bpm by arrival in the OR or within 9 minutes (often the same interval due to transport), the decision for immediate delivery should be revisited.

Sinusoidal pattern: A regular oscillation of baseline long-term variability resembling a sine wave. This undulating pattern, lasting at least 10 minutes, has a relatively fixed period of 3–5 cycles/minute and amplitude of 5–15 beats/minute above and below the baseline. The cycles are round and baseline variability otherwise absent. There are several opiates known to be associated with a pseudo-sinudoidal pattern. A true sinusoidal pattern is associated with fetal anemia and high rates of fetal morbidity and mortality (Figure 5.8).[26]

Contraction pattern: Never forget the "bottom line." Note the duration of contractions and the interval between contractions. Describe the contraction pattern in terms of the number of contractions in a 10-minute window, rather than the time between contractions. Identify the presence of tachysystole (more than 5 contractions per 10-minute window averaged over 30 continuous minutes), or frequent, low-amplitude, high-baseline contractions in association with a suspicious FHR pattern that may be suggestive of placental abruption.

NICHD recommended categories

Because of widespread interpretation inconsistency,[27,28,29] the American College of Obstetricians and Gynecologists (ACOG), the Society for Maternal-Fetal Medicine (SMFM), and the United States National Institute of Child Health and Human Development (NICHD) jointly endorsed a three-category system for intrapartum EFM based on "expert opinion" (Table 5.2). In one study of intrapartum tracings from 48,000 singleton, non-anomalous fetuses, Category I patterns were observed in over 99% of tracings, Category II patterns were observed at some point in 84% of tracings, and Category III patterns were observed at some point in 0.1% of tracings.[30] Throughout labor, the pattern was Category I about 78% of the time, Category II, 22% of the time, and Category III, 0.004% of the time. The definitions are as follows:

Table 5.2 NICHD three-category fetal heart rate interpretation classification

Category I
Category I fetal heart rate (FHR) tracings include all of the following:
- Baseline rate: 110–160 beats per minute (bpm)
- Baseline FHR variability: moderate
- Late or variable decelerations: absent
- Early decelerations: present or absent
- Accelerations: present or absent

Category II
Category II FHR tracings include all FHR tracings not categorized as Category I or Category III. Examples include any of the following:
Baseline rate
- Bradycardia not accompanied by absent baseline variability
- Tachycardia

Baseline FHR variability
- Minimal baseline variability
- Absent baseline variability not accompanied by recurrent decelerations
- Marked baseline variability

Accelerations
- Absence of spontaneous or induced accelerations after fetal stimulation
- Periodic or episodic decelerations
- Recurrent variable decelerations accompanied by minimal or moderate baseline variability

Table 5.2 (*cont.*)

- Prolonged deceleration >2 minutes but <10 minutes
- Recurrent late decelerations with moderate baseline variability
- Variable decelerations with atypical characteristics, such as slow return to baseline

Category III

Include either:

- Absent baseline FHR variability and any of the following:
  - Recurrent late decelerations
  - Recurrent variable decelerations
  - Bradycardia
- Sinusoidal pattern

(Modified from reference 12)

Category I tracings

A Category I tracing is defined as:

- baseline rate: 110–160 bpm
- moderate baseline FHR variability (amplitude 6–25 bpm)
- no recurrent late or variable decelerations
- early decelerations may be present or absent
- accelerations may be present or absent.

Category I patterns are considered "normal" since studies reveal these patterns predict absence of significant fetal metabolic acidemia at the time of observation.[31,32,33,34] No intervention is indicated.

If the maternal and fetal conditions appear stable, it is reasonable to stop a Category I tracing for up to 30 minutes to allow for ambulation, bathing, or position changes. For pregnancies at low risk of developing intrapartum fetal acidosis, the ACOG recommends the tracing be reviewed at least every 30 minutes during the 1st stage of labor, and every 15 minutes during the 2nd stage.[35] We suggest making a note in the medical record stating the interpretation and plan to document each EFM review. For patients with pregnancy complications (e.g., fetal growth restriction, pre-eclampsia), where the risk of developing intrapartum fetal acidosis is higher, the tracing should be reviewed at least every 15 minutes in the 1st stage of labor and every 5 minutes during the 2nd stage.

Category III tracings

A Category III tracing is defined by the following criteria:

- Absent baseline FHR variability *and* any of the following:
  recurrent late decelerations

  recurrent variable decelerations

  bradycardia

or

- A sinusoidal pattern.

In practice, this definition has been problematic because observers frequently disagree on whether there is absent or minimal variability.[29,36] Thus the proposed management covers both minimal and absent variability. A Category III tracing is associated with an increased risk of fetal hypoxic acidemia, which can cause CP and neonatal hypoxic ischemic encephalopathy. It is hypothesized, but remains to be proven, that the detection of fetal decompensation and timely and effective intervention(s) before the acidosis becomes severe can prevent CP as well as perinatal/neonatal morbidity or mortality. This is likely true only for acute events in contrast to chronic hypoxia during the antepartum period. Preparations for delivery and the initiation of resuscitative measures to improve uteroplacental perfusion and oxygen delivery should be made with a Category III pattern.[37,38,39,40] Cesarean delivery may be avoided if *in utero* resuscitation corrects the Category III tracing.

Scalp stimulation to provoke FHR acceleration from baseline may be useful if fetal scalp sampling is not practiced. The probability of at least a mild fetal acidosis is less than 10% when scalp stimulation causes an acceleration compared to about 50% when no acceleration occurs in this setting. Delivery should be expedited if scalp stimulation fails to generate an acceleration and there is no improvement in the FHR tracing after resuscitative measures. The time from decision to delivery must consider the health of both the mother and fetus: there may be circumstances (e.g., difficult maternal airway, maternal coagulopathy, severe obesity) where safe delivery cannot be performed expeditiously.

In utero resuscitation

The following general measures for the management of Category III tracings are aimed at improving uteroplacental perfusion and maternal/fetal oxygenation (Table 5.3).

- Reposition the patient onto her side (left or right); changing the maternal position may both reduce any cord compression and improve maternal blood flow to the placenta.

Table 5.3 Possible intrauterine resuscitative measures for Category II and/or Category III tracings

Goal	Associated FHR abnormality	Potential intervention(s)
Promote fetal oxygenation and improve uteroplacental blood flow	■ Recurrent late decelerations ■ Prolonged decelerations or bradycardia ■ Minimal or absent FHR variability	Place mother in a lateral position (either left or right) Administer oxygen Give IV fluid bolus Reduce uterine contraction frequency
Reduce uterine activity	■ Tachysystole with Category II or III tracing	Discontinue oxytocin or cervical ripening agents Administer tocolytic medication (e.g., terbutaline)
Alleviate umbilical cord compression	■ Recurrent variable decelerations ■ Prolonged decelerations or bradycardia	Reposition mother (left or right lateral, hands and knees) Perform amnio-infusion If umbilical cord prolapse is noted, elevate the presenting fetal part while preparing for operative delivery

(Simpson K R, James D C. Efficacy of intrauterine resuscitation techniques in improving fetal oxygen status during labor. Obstet Gynecol 2005; 105:1362.)

■ Administer an IV fluid bolus (e.g., 500 to 1,000 ml of lactated Ringer's or normal saline solution). A fluid bolus may improve placental blood flow, and thus fetal oxygenation, if the patient is hypovolemic due to insufficient oral or intravenous intake, vomiting, or sympathetic blockade. Fluids should be given cautiously in women at increased risk of volume overload (e.g., pre-eclampsia, cardiac disease, or receiving beta-adrenergic tocolytic agents).

■ The administration of maternal oxygen (e.g., 8 to 10 l/minute of oxygen via non-rebreather mask) in response to a Category II or III tracing is practiced in many countries including North America. There are no adequately powered studies to conclude the practice actually improves outcomes, and only laboratory studies revealing increased fetal oxygen levels with maternal hyperoxygenation, and antedotal reports of late decelerations resolving with oxygen and then returning when the oxygen was discontinued.[41] It has even been suggested that maternal hyperoxygenation poses a risk to mother and child.[42] It is important to remember that if giving oxygen, pregnant women are characteristically mouth breathers due to pregnancy mediated swelling of the nasal mucosa.

- Discontinue uterotonic drugs.

- Consider administering a tocolytic drug (e.g., terbutaline 250 mcg subcutaneously) to prolong the interval for uninterrupted placental perfusion.

- Should the patient have recently received epidural medication for labor pain, ask the anesthesia team to evaluate the patient for administration of an alpha-adrenergic agonist (e.g., phenylephrine, ephedrine) to reduce sympathetic blockade.

- If there are variable decelerations, consider an amnio-infusion.

Although improved delivery of oxygen to the fetal tissues may be beneficial in some cases, the underlying causes of fetal hypoxemia need to be addressed, as fetal acidemia will not be corrected by maternal oxygen administration alone.[42]

Category II tracings

Category II tracings include all FHR patterns neither classified as Category I (normal) nor Category III (abnormal). The Society of Obstetricians and Gynaecologists of Canada (SOGC) classify such tracings as "atypical."[43]

The potential for fetal acidosis varies greatly across the different types of Category II tracings, and some investigators have proposed a five-tier FHR classification system, which may better define fetuses at increased risk of acidosis.[44,45,46] Like the NICHD three-tier system, there is currently no evidence that the additional subgroups actually improve the predictive accuracy for acidemia.

Patients with Category II tracings should be evaluated for factors that may reduce fetal oxygenation, taking into account clinical circumstances (e.g., trial of labor after a previous cesarean delivery, IUGR associated with abnormal Doppler studies, abruption, etc.), and the stage and progress of labor (Figure 5.9). Resuscitative measures should follow those described for minimal variability. Continue continuous surveillance and frequent reassessment until the pattern resolves or progresses to Category III. Ancillary tests can be performed to gain more information, but there is no standard evaluation. In general, FHR accelerations are highly predictive of normal fetal acid–base status and provide reassurance that expeditious delivery is unnecessary.

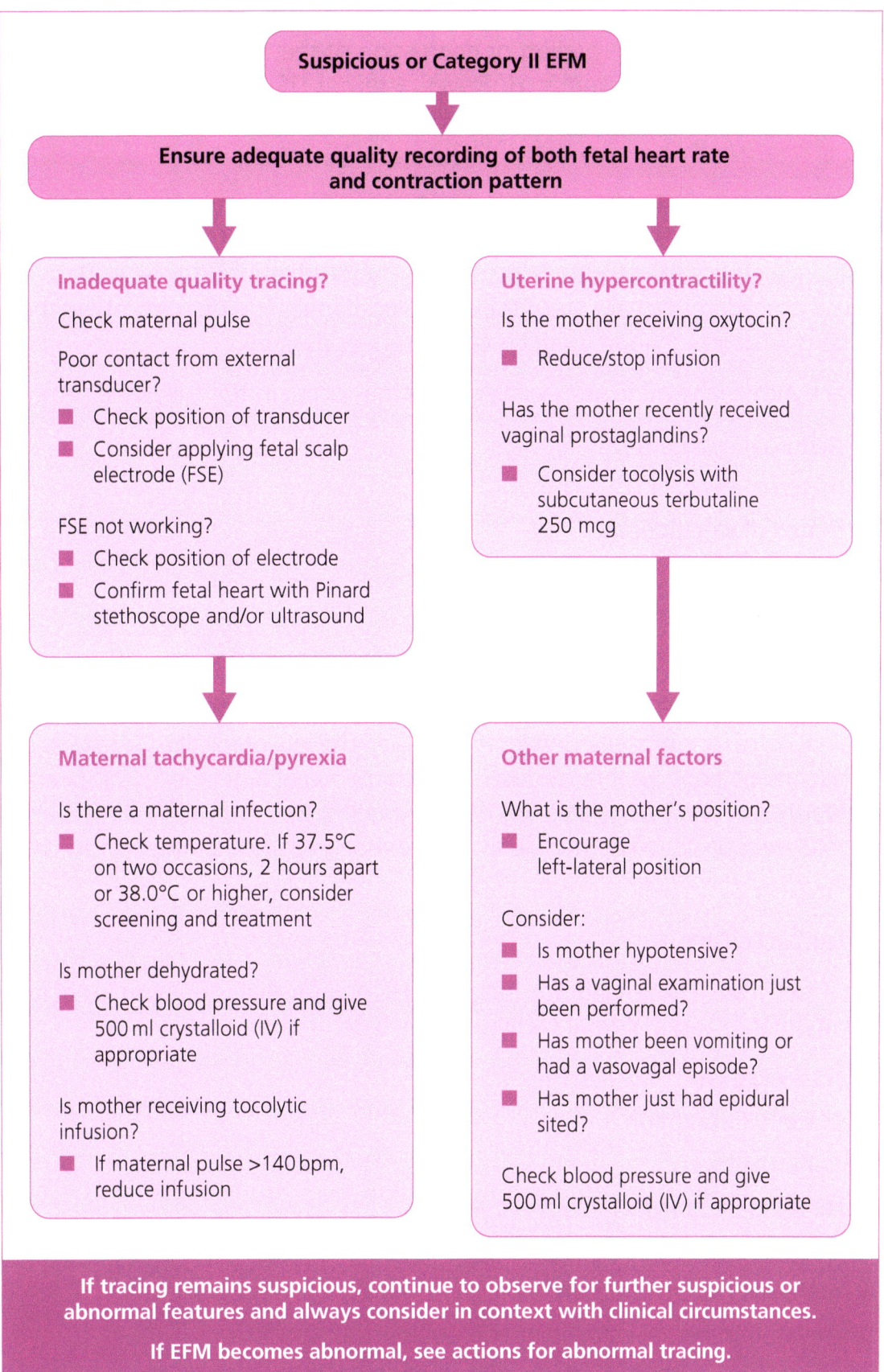

Suspicious or Category II EFM

Ensure adequate quality recording of both fetal heart rate and contraction pattern

Inadequate quality tracing?

Check maternal pulse

Poor contact from external transducer?
- Check position of transducer
- Consider applying fetal scalp electrode (FSE)

FSE not working?
- Check position of electrode
- Confirm fetal heart with Pinard stethoscope and/or ultrasound

Uterine hypercontractility?

Is the mother receiving oxytocin?
- Reduce/stop infusion

Has the mother recently received vaginal prostaglandins?
- Consider tocolysis with subcutaneous terbutaline 250 mcg

Maternal tachycardia/pyrexia

Is there a maternal infection?
- Check temperature. If 37.5°C on two occasions, 2 hours apart or 38.0°C or higher, consider screening and treatment

Is mother dehydrated?
- Check blood pressure and give 500 ml crystalloid (IV) if appropriate

Is mother receiving tocolytic infusion?
- If maternal pulse >140 bpm, reduce infusion

Other maternal factors

What is the mother's position?
- Encourage left-lateral position

Consider:
- Is mother hypotensive?
- Has a vaginal examination just been performed?
- Has mother been vomiting or had a vasovagal episode?
- Has mother just had epidural sited?

Check blood pressure and give 500 ml crystalloid (IV) if appropriate

If tracing remains suspicious, continue to observe for further suspicious or abnormal features and always consider in context with clinical circumstances.

If EFM becomes abnormal, see actions for abnormal tracing.

Figure 5.9 Suggested actions if EFM suspicious

The STAN fetal heart monitor measures the fetal electrocardiogram (EKG) during labor to detect elevation or depression of the ST segment, which is suggestive of fetal hypoxemia. However, a recent US randomized controlled trial (RCT) concluded that there was no advantage of STAN over traditional visual methods.[47]

Fetal scalp blood sampling for pH or lactate level is no longer performed in most labor and delivery units because of a general lack of training in US residency programs, despite its proven ability for diagnosing fetal acidosis. These procedures remain an option in skilled hands. The discomfort for the patient is far less than an unnecessary cesarean delivery.

Fetal hypoxia leading to late decelerations may occur in the following settings:

- maternal hypotension
- maternal hypoxia
- maternal vasculopathy
- maternal fever
- uterine tachysystole
- placental disorders associated with placental dysfunction.

The assessment of FHR variability and accelerations should be part of the evaluation of recurrent late decelerations, given the low predictive value of late decelerations alone for fetal acidosis and poor neonatal outcome.[48,49] Moderate variability is strongly associated (98%) with an umbilical artery pH >7.15,[50] and spontaneous or elicited FHR accelerations are strongly associated with pH >7.10.[37]

Fetal tachycardia

Fetal tachycardia is defined as a baseline FHR greater than 160 bpm for at least 10 minutes. Causes of fetal tachycardia include:

- fetal hypoxia
- placental abruption
- maternal fever
- maternal–fetal infection
- medications (e.g., beta-agonists, atropine, cocaine)
- maternal hyperthyroidism
- elevated maternal catecholamine levels.

Fetal tachycardia may rarely be due to tachyarrhythmias. Such tachyarrhythmias are characterized by a high FHR, often greater than 200 bpm. The fetal capacity to acutely alter stroke volume of the heart is limited. As the rate increases, filling time and ultimately cardiac output decreases. A fetal tachycardia below 200 bpm alone is not strongly associated with fetal acidemia, unless associated with recurrent decelerations, absent accelerations, or minimal/absent variability.[51,52] The latter can be misleading as the increase in rate alone decreases the opportunity for variability by shortening the time between beats. Appropriate treatment should be initiated if a cause can be identified (e.g., administer acetaminophen for fever). An expedited delivery is indicated if acidemia or placental abruption is suspected. Tachycardia due to chorioamnionitis is generally not an indication for expedited delivery unless there is a Category III tracing, or the patient is remote from delivery and the tachycardia is unresolved by hydration and acetaminophen.

Variable decelerations with variability and or accelerations

Variable decelerations occur when the umbilical cord is compressed. Intermittent variable decelerations (associated with <50% of contractions) are common intrapartum and typically associated with moderate variability and/or accelerations. There are only three possibilities when there is a vulnerable cord: it can get better, worse, or stay the same. Such variable decelerations do not require intervention.

A mixed metabolic/respiratory acidosis or ultimately a pure metabolic acidosis can develop with increasing duration, depth, and frequency of variable decelerations, and recurrent variable decelerations (>50% of contractions) require close surveillance for loss of variability and accelerations.

Resuscitative measures focus on relieving the cord compression. Change of maternal position is a reasonable first option and an amnio-infusion a reasonable second-line option. Amnio-infusion reduces the risk of progressive cord compression later in the labor, reducing FHR abnormalities by almost 60% compared to controls.[53] There is also a significant reduction in the number of cesarean deliveries for FHR abnormalities and an improvement in several neonatal outcomes, including fewer umbilical artery <7.20 pH measurements (though the lower limit of normal after labor is approximately pH 7.12). Delivery is indicated if a Category III tracing develops.

Loss of variability without decelerations

The new onset of minimal variability (amplitude 1 to 5 bpm) may occur for several reasons, including:

- fetal sleep cycle – quiet sleep generally lasts approximately 20 minutes at term, but may persist for as long as an hour
- CNS depressants – common medications that reduce variability include opioids and magnesium sulfate. The effect of maternal opioids on FHR variability generally lasts no more than two hours
- fetal hypoxemia.

A reasonable approach to new onset minimal fetal variability if the FHR pattern has been normal and there are no decelerations is to make a presumptive diagnosis of a fetal sleep cycle or the effect of recently administered maternal medications. It is reasonable to try to induce accelerations with scalp stimulation, as the presence of accelerations is strong evidence for the absence of fetal acidemia at that time.[37] A fluid bolus or repositioning are also considered appropriate measures but have little objective study for support. Long-standing loss of variability may reflect congenital or acquired anomalies of the CNS or heart, or very pre term gestation.[54,55,56]

Fetal bradycardia/prolonged deceleration without loss of variability

Prolonged decelerations or fetal bradycardia (below 110 bpm) are approached similarly, since the distinction between these two is based on the number of minutes the decrease in FHR persists. The causes of prolonged deceleration or fetal bradycardia include:

- rapid fetal descent
- umbilical cord prolapse
- placental abruption
- maternal hypotension
- uterine rupture
- tachysystole.

Fetal acidemia is unlikely when the FHR returns to a normal baseline rate and variability and accelerations are present.

Treatment of fetal bradycardia or prolonged deceleration is directed at the cause. Evaluation should include assessment of maternal blood pressure and contraction frequency and strength, and physical examination for evidence of rapid fetal descent, cord prolapse, placental abruption, or uterine rupture. Terbutaline may be used to treat tachysystole (250 mcg SQ). Side effects of terbutaline include maternal tachycardia (palpitations) and fetal tachycardia, increased blood pressure, tremor, nausea, nervousness, and dizziness.

Delivery is indicated when resuscitative measures are not possible or fails to resolve the bradycardia. In a study of 5,300 term, healthy singleton pregnancies at full dilation in cephalic presentation, a terminal deceleration occurred in 17.7% and only 1.3% had an umbilical arterial pH <7.10.[55] Of the 31 fetuses with a terminal bradycardia (FHR <110 bpm for ≥10 minutes before delivery), only 4 had an umbilical arterial pH ≤7.10. Although infants with terminal bradycardia had an increased risk of acidemia, the positive predictive value approximates 1 in 7. The authors noted the umbilical artery pH declined about 0.04 units for every two minutes after the first two minutes. This is consistent with earlier studies noting the umbilical artery pH declines by 0.03 pH units per minute of complete cord occlusion (assumed to be the case when the FHR is less than 90 bpm). An expedited delivery is indicated should a Category III tracing develop.

Expedite delivery

- The urgency and mode of delivery should take into account the severity of the fetal heart rate abnormality and the clinical circumstances.
- The accepted standard is that birth should be accomplished within 30 minutes of the decision.

Continuous EFM in the presence of oxytocin

A full assessment by an experienced labor nurse, midwife, or obstetrician should be performed and documented in the labor notes before initiating an oxytocin infusion. The rate may be increased until the woman is experiencing four or five contractions every 10 minutes. The infusion rate should be reduced if more than five contractions occur in 10 minutes over a period of 30 minutes. An experienced obstetrician should review the FHR pattern when oxytocin is indicated or infusing, and the tracing is thought to be either Category II or III. Once reviewed, the obstetrician may recommend the oxytocin continue to be increased but only to a dose that achieves four to five contractions in 10 minutes.[15]

The oxytocin infusion should be stopped if the FHR pattern progresses to a Category III. If warranted, oxytocin may be cautiously restarted if the Category III pattern resolves.

Newborn assessment

The Apgar score need for intubation and abnormal behavior are important components of the newborn assessment. Yet they are subjective, and by themselves are not indicative of asphyxia. Asphyxia is defined in the perinatal period as the combination of hypoxia and acidosis with impaired organ function (tissue acidemia).[57] As a result, both clinical and biochemical information are required to differentiate between an asphyxiated infant and one that is depressed for other reasons (infection, congenital abnormalities, maternal analgesia, etc.). If not collected routinely, paired umbilical artery and vein blood samples should be collected to provide an objective outcome measure whenever:

- an urgent or emergency cesarean section is performed
- an operative vaginal delivery is performed
- a shoulder dystocia has occurred
- the Apgar score at 5 minutes is 6 or less.

The umbilical acid–base status at birth can be important for medico-legal reasons and for risk management strategies.[58] Clamped cord segments or blood stored in syringes can be left at room temperature for up to 60 minutes without significant changes in pH or CO_2.[59,60]

Antenatal FHR interpretation

A review in the *Cochrane Database of Systematic Reviews* neither confirmed nor refuted any benefit of routine EFM of "at risk" women, as the evidence for EFM use antenatally is based on a few small studies from the 1980s (four trials enrolling 1588 women in total).[61]

In clinical practice, there are a variety of antenatal indications for EFM after 23 to 24 weeks. The presence of a normal fetal heart rate pattern (i.e., showing accelerations of fetal heart rate coinciding with fetal movements) is indicative of a fetus with a properly functioning autonomic nervous system that is inconsistent with a significant fetal acidosis.

The nomenclature for the reading of antepartum tracings should be the same as that used intrapartum. Keep in mind it is normal to have occasional small decelerations associated with fetal movement or Braxton Hicks contractions in preterm fetuses. The FHR baseline typically declines with advancing gestational age and variability increase. Sleep–wake cycles become more distinct and the switch between states well demarcated. It is also important to remember that the reason for performing antenatal EFM is relevant when determining any action to be taken, as is the gestation and the status of the membranes. When an abnormal FHR pattern is identified, it should be reviewed by an obstetrician as soon as possible (within 30 minutes) to make a clear action plan that may include:

- other tests to be performed (ultrasound scan for growth, Doppler studies, etc.)
- a specified time for the next obstetric review
- consideration of any need for an expedited delivery.

References

1. elearning for health. RCOG/RCM EFM training package. 2011.

2. Nelson KB, Blair E.Prenatal factors in singletons with cerebral palsy born at or near term.*N Engl J Med*. 2015; 373: 946–53.

3. Nelson KB, Willoughby RE. Infection, inflammation, and the risk of cerebral palsy. *Curr Opin Neurol* 2000; 13: 133–9.

4. Grant A. Monitoring the fetus during labour. In Chalmers I, Enkin M, Keirse MC (eds) *A Guide to Effective Care in Pregnancy and Childbirth*. Oxford: Oxford University Press; 1989. pp. 846–82.

5. Thacker SB, Stroup D, Chang M.Continuous electronic heart rate monitoring for fetal assessment during labor. *Cochrane Database Syst Rev* 2001; 2: CD000063.

6. MacDonald D, Grant A, Sheridan-Pereira M, Boylan P, Chalmers I. The Dublin randomized controlled trial of intrapartum fetal heart rate monitoring. *Am J Obstet Gynecol* 1985; 152: 524–39.

7. Murphy KW, Johnson P, Moorcraft J, Pattison R, Russell V, Turnbull A. Birth asphyxia and the intrapartum cardiotocograph. *Br J Obstet Gynaecol* 1990; 97: 470–9.

8. Confidential Enquiry into Stillbirths and Deaths in Infancy. *4th Annual Report*. London: Maternal and Child Health Research Consortium; 1997.

9. Confidential Enquiry into Stillbirths and Deaths in Infancy. *5th Annual Report*. London: Maternal and Child Health Research Consortium; 1998.

10. Confidential Enquiry into Stillbirths and Deaths in Infancy. *7th Annual Report*. London: Maternal and Child Health Research Consortium; 2001.

11. West Midlands Perinatal Audit. *Stillbirth and Neonatal Death 1991–1994. Report of National, Regional, District and Unit Mortality Rates*. Keele: West Midlands Perinatal Audit; 1996.

12. Macones GA, Hankins GD, Spong CY, Hauth J, Moore T. The 2008 National Institute of Child Health and Human Development workshop report on electronic fetal monitoring: update on definitions, interpretation, and research guidelines. *Obstet Gynecol* 2008; 112: 661–6.

13. Clements RV, Simanowitz A. Cerebral palsy: the international consensus statement. *Clin Risk* 2000; 6: 135–6.

14. Pickering J. Legal comment on the international consensus statement on causation of cerebral palsy. *Clin Risk* 2000; 6: 143–4.

15. Symonds EM. Litigation and birth related injuries. In Chamberlain G (ed.) *How to Avoid Medico-legal Problems in Obstetrics and Gynaecology*. London: Chameleon Press; 1991.

16. Berglund S, Pettersson H, Cnattingius S, Grunewald C. How often is a low Apgar score the result of substandard care during labour? *BJOG* 2010; 117: 968–78.

17. The NHS Litigation Authority. Factsheet 3: Information on claims. London: NHSLA; 2011 [www.nhsla.com].

18. NHS Litigation Authority. *Clinical Negligence Scheme for Trusts Maternity Clinical Risk Management Standards*. London: NHSLA; 2011 [www.nhsla.com/RiskManagement].

19. Draycott T, Sibanda T, Owen L, Akande V, Winter C, Reading S, *et al.* Does training in obstetric emergencies improve neonatal outcome? *BJOG* 2006; 113: 177–82.

20. MacEachin SR, Lopez CM, Powell KJ, Corbett NL. The fetal heart rate collaborative practice project: situational awareness in electronic fetal monitoring: a Kaiser Permanente Perinatal Patient Safety Program Initiative. *J Perinat Neonatal Nurs* 2009; 23: 314–23.

21. Pehrson C, Sorensen J, Amer-Wåhlin I. Evaluation and impact of cardiotocography training programmes: a systematic review. *BJOG* 2011; 118: 926–35.

22. Lagercrantz H, Bistoletti P. Catecholamine release in the newborn infant at birth. *Pediatr Res* 1977; 11: 889–93.

23. Map of Medicine. Evidence summary for the first stage of labour. International. 2011 [http://eng.mapofmedicine.com/evidence/map/normal_birth1.html].

24. Herbert WN, Stuart NN, Butler LS. Electronic fetal heart rate monitoring with intrauterine fetal demise. *J Obstet Gynecol Neonatal Nurs* 1987; 16: 249–52.

25. Maeder HP, Lippert TH. Misinterpretation of heart rate recordings in fetal death. *Eur J Obstet Gynecol* 1972; 6: 167–70.

26. Schneider EP, Tropper PJ. The variable deceleration, prolonged deceleration, and sinusoidal fetal heart rate. *Clin Obstet Gynecol* 1986; 29: 64–72.

27. Nielsen PV, Stigsby B, Nickelsen C, Nim J. Intra- and inter-observer variability in the assessment of intrapartum cardiotocograms. *Acta Obstet Gynecol Scand* 1987; 66: 421.

28. Beaulieu MD, Fabia J, Leduc B, *et al.* The reproducibility of intrapartum cardiotocogram assessments. *Can Med Assoc J* 1982; 127: 214.

29. Chauhan SP, Klauser CK, Woodring TC, *et al.* Intrapartum nonreassuring fetal heart rate tracing and prediction of adverse outcomes: interobserver variability. *Am J Obstet Gynecol* 2008; 199: 623.e1.

30. Jackson M, Holmgren CM, Esplin MS, *et al.* Frequency of fetal heart rate categories and short-term neonatal outcome. *Obstet Gynecol* 2011; 118: 803.

31. Berkus MD, Langer O, Samueloff A, *et al.* Electronic fetal monitoring: what's reassuring? *Acta Obstet Gynecol Scand* 1999; 78: 15.

32. Krebs HB, Petres RE, Dunn LJ, Smith PJ. Intrapartum fetal heart rate monitoring. VI. Prognostic significance of accelerations. *Am J Obstet Gynecol* 1982; 142: 297.

33. Tejani N, Mann LI, Bhakthavathsalan A, Weiss RR. Correlation of fetal heart rate-uterine contraction patterns with fetal scalp blood pH. *Obstet Gynecol* 1975; 46: 392.

34. Dellinger EH, Boehm FH, Crane MM. Electronic fetal heart rate monitoring: early neonatal outcomes associated with normal rate, fetal stress, and fetal distress. *Am J Obstet Gynecol* 2000; 182: 214.

35. American College of Obstetricians and Gynecologists. ACOG Practice Bulletin No. 106: Intrapartum fetal heart rate monitoring: nomenclature, interpretation, and general management principles. *Obstet Gynecol* 2009; 114: 192.

36. Blackwell SC, Grobman WA, Antoniewicz L, *et al.* Interobserver and intraobserver reliability of the NICHD 3-Tier Fetal Heart Rate Interpretation System. *Am J Obstet Gynecol* 2011; 205: 378.e1.

37. Skupski DW, Rosenberg CR, Eglinton GS. Intrapartum fetal stimulation tests: a meta-analysis. *Obstet Gynecol* 2002; 99: 129.

38. Fawole B, Hofmeyr GJ. Maternal oxygen administration for fetal distress. *Cochrane Database Syst Rev* 2012; 12: CD000136.

39. Simpson KR. Intrauterine resuscitation during labor: review of current methods and supportive evidence. *J Midwifery Womens Health* 2007; 52: 229.

40. Simpson KR, James DC. Efficacy of intrauterine resuscitation techniques in improving fetal oxygen status during labor. *Obstet Gynecol* 2005; 105: 1362.

41. Garite TJ, Nageotte MP, Parer JT. Should we really avoid giving oxygen to mothers with concerning fetal heart rate patterns? *Am J Obstet Gynecol* 2015; 212: 459–60.

42. Hamel MS, Anderson BL, Rouse DJ. Oxygen for intrauterine resuscitation: of unproved benefit and potentially harmful. *Am J Obstet Gynecol* 2014; 211: 124.

43. Liston R, Sawchuck D, Young D, *et al.* Fetal health surveillance: antepartum and intrapartum consensus guideline. *J Obstet Gynaecol Can* 2007; 29: S3.

44. Coletta J, Murphy E, Rubeo Z, Gyamfi-Bannerman C. The 5-tier system of assessing fetal heart rate tracings is superior to the 3-tier system in identifying fetal acidemia. *Am J Obstet Gynecol* 2012; 206: 226.e1.

45. Gyamfi Bannerman C, Grobman WA, Antoniewicz L, *et al.* Assessment of the concordance among 2-tier, 3-tier, and 5-tier fetal heart rate classification systems. *Am J Obstet Gynecol* 2011; 205: 288.e1.

46. Sadaka A, Furuhashi M, Minami H, *et al.* Observation on validity of the five-tier system for fetal heart rate pattern interpretation proposed by Japan Society of Obstetricians and Gynecologists. *J Matern Fetal Neonatal Med* 2011; 24: 1465.

47. Saade GS for the NICHD MFMU Network. Fetal ECG analysis of the ST segment as an adjunct to intrapartum fetal heart rate monitoring: a randomized clinical trial. *Am J Obstet Gynecol* 2015; 212: S2.

48. Nelson KB, Dambrosia JM, Ting TY, Grether JK. Uncertain value of electronic fetal monitoring in predicting cerebral palsy. *N Engl J Med* 1996; 334: 613.

49. Larma JD, Silva AM, Holcroft CJ, *et al.* Intrapartum electronic fetal heart rate monitoring and the identification of metabolic acidosis and hypoxic-ischemic encephalopathy. *Am J Obstet Gynecol* 2007; 197: 301.e1.

50. Parer JT, King T, Flanders S, *et al.* Fetal acidemia and electronic fetal heart rate patterns: is there evidence of an association? *J Matern Fetal Neonatal Med* 2006; 19: 289.

51. Honjo S, Yamaguchi M. Umbilical artery blood acid–base analysis and fetal heart rate baseline in the second stage of labor. *J Obstet Gynaecol Res* 2001; 27: 249.

52. Strachan BK, Sahota DS, van Wijngaarden WJ, *et al.* Computerised analysis of the fetal heart rate and relation to acidaemia at delivery. *BJOG* 2001; 108: 848.

53. Hofmeyr GJ, Lawrie TA. Amnioinfusion for potential or suspected umbilical cord compression in labour. *Cochrane Database Syst Rev* 2012; 1: CD000013.

54. Assali NS, Brinkman CR 3rd, Woods JR Jr, *et al.* Development of neuro-humoral control of fetal, neonatal, and adult cardiovascular functions. *Am J Obstet Gynecol* 1977; 129: 748.

55. van der Moer PE, Gerretsen G, Visser GH. Fixed fetal heart rate pattern after intrauterine accidental decerebration. *Obstet Gynecol* 1985; 65: 125.

56. Cahill AG, Caughey AB, Roehl KA, *et al.* Terminal fetal heart decelerations and neonatal outcomes. *Obstet Gynecol* 2013; 122: 1070.

57. Greene KR, Rosen KG. Intrapartum asphyxia. In Levene MI, Lilford R (eds) *Fetal and Neonatal Neurology and Neurosurgery, 2nd edn*. Edinburgh: Churchill Livingstone; 1995, pp. 389–404.

58. MacLennan A. A template for defining a causal relation between acute intrapartum events and cerebral palsy: international consensus statement. *BMJ* 1999; 319: 1054–9.

59. Duerbeck NB, Chaffin DG, Seeds JW. A practical approach to umbilical artery pH and blood gas determinations. *Obstet Gynecol* 1992; 79: 959–62.

60. Sykes GS, Molloy PM. Effects of delays in collection or analysis on the results of umbilical cord blood measurements. *Br J Obstet Gynaecol* 1984; 91: 989–92.

61. Pattison N, McCowan L. Cardiotocography for antepartum fetal assessment. *Cochrane Database Syst Rev* 2000; 2: CD001068.

Module 6
Pre-eclampsia and eclampsia

Key learning points

- Understand the risk factors for and recognize the signs and symptoms of severe pre-eclampsia.
- Understand the potential complications of severe hypertension (systolic blood pressure $\geq$160 mmHg) and its management.
- Manage an eclamptic seizure effectively.
- Understand the care and monitoring required for a woman being treated with magnesium sulfate.
- The importance of detailed contemporaneous documentation.

Common difficulties observed in training drills

- Not stating the problem clearly when help arrives.
- Not involving an experienced obstetrician and anesthesiologist in the management of women with severe pre-eclampsia and eclampsia.
- Failing to adequately treat hypertension in a timely fashion.
- Incorrect administration or labeling of magnesium sulfate.
- Failing to restrict fluids.
- Failing to stabilize the woman before delivery.
- Forgetting to perform basic resuscitation.

Introduction

Hypertensive disorders are the second most common cause of maternal death worldwide.[1] A total of 297 women in the United States died during the five-year period between 2006 and 2010 from complications of pre-eclampsia or eclampsia. Another 207 women died from cerebrovascular accidents, with most being associated with hypertensive disease.[2] While the overall rate of death in the United States from pre-eclampsia/eclampsia has been roughly halved since 1987, the rate of cerebrovascular accidents has steadily increased. In contrast, only 19 women in the UK died between 2006 and 2008 as a direct result of pre-eclampsia or eclampsia; about one quarter of the US rate.[3] An additional three women died as a result of acute fatty liver of pregnancy, which is thought to be a "pre-eclampsia spectrum" disease. All UK maternal mortalities were reviewed in detail, and the care of 20 of the 22 women was judged substandard. While direct deaths from pre-eclampsia/eclampsia are at an all-time low, 14 of the 22 were considered preventable. Intracranial hemorrhage was the single largest cause of death and indicates a failure of effective antihypertensive therapy.[3,4] Severe hypertension (systolic blood pressure >160 mmHg) must be treated to prevent maternal mortality and morbidity.[5]

Pre-eclampsia

Pre-eclampsia is a multisystem syndrome unique to pregnancy characterized by new-onset hypertension with significant new-onset proteinuria after 20 weeks.[4] It occurs in about 3% of pregnancies and at a rate 1.5- to 2-fold higher in first pregnancies. Pre-eclampsia is a disorder of endothelial function specific to pregnancy that is thought triggered by an abnormality of placental implantation. The US rates of pre-eclampsia and severe pre-eclampsia have increased over the past few decades, driven in part by the rising rates of obesity.[6] In addition to maternal mortality, pre-eclampsia is one of the most common underlying causes of maternal morbidity and perinatal morbidity/mortality (Box 6.1 and 6.2).

Predisposing risk factors for pre-eclampsia are shown in Box 6.3.

Eclampsia

Eclampsia is defined as one or more convulsions in a woman with pre-eclampsia and complicates 2 to 3% of patients with severe pre-eclampsia. However, a significant proportion of women who have an eclamptic seizure do not have established hypertension and proteinuria before their first eclamptic

Box 6.1 Maternal complications of pre-eclampsia

- Intracranial hemorrhage (a leading cause of death from severe pre-eclampsia)
- Placental abruption
- Eclampsia
- Atypical pre-eclampsia, aka HELLP syndrome (hemolysis, elevated liver enzymes, and low platelets)
- Disseminated intravascular coagulation
- Renal failure
- Pulmonary edema
- Acute respiratory distress syndrome (ARDS)
- Peripartum cardiomyopathy

Box 6.2 Fetal complications of pre-eclampsia

- Early-onset fetal growth restriction
- Oligohydramnios
- Hypoxia from placental dysfunction
- Placental abruption
- Preterm birth

seizure.[7] Forty-four percent of seizures occur postpartum, 38% antepartum and 18% intrapartum. The seizure recurrence rate is 5 to 30% even with adequate treatment. While the rate of eclampsia in the United States has been stable,[8] there is a high rate of maternal complications, with at least one major morbidity in 10% of eclamptic women.[5] Perinatal mortality associated with eclampsia is reportedly 10 times that of normal pregnancies.[5]

Presenting features

Eclampsia presents as generalized seizures, with jerking limb and head movements. The mother may become cyanotic, and tongue biting or urinary

> **Box 6.3 Predisposing risk factors for pre-eclampsia**
>
> ■ Nulliparity
> ■ Hypertensive disease during a previous pregnancy
> ■ Chronic hypertension
> ■ Family history of pre-eclampsia
> ■ Pre-existing diabetes
> ■ Multiple pregnancy
> ■ Obesity
> ■ Extremes of maternal age
> ■ Autoimmune disease (e.g., systemic lupus erythematous, antiphospholipid syndrome)
> ■ Renal disease
> ■ 10 or more years since the last pregnancy

incontinence may also occur. Most seizures are single and self-limited and resolve within 90 seconds. Eclampsia can be a very frightening experience for both family members and staff.

Management of eclampsia

The management of eclampsia involves basic life support as well as seizure management. An outline for the initial management of eclampsia is shown in Figure 6.1. Management is described in more detail in the next section and is followed by details for severe pre-eclampsia. Guidelines for the treatment of hypertension are provided in the final section.

Call for help

Activate the emergency call button to summon help. This includes calling for the senior labor nurse, the most experienced obstetrician available, an anesthesiologist, and additional nurses and maternity nursing assistants to provide clinical support and document actions.

■ Note the time the seizure occurred and its duration.
■ Note the time of the emergency call and time of arrival of staff.

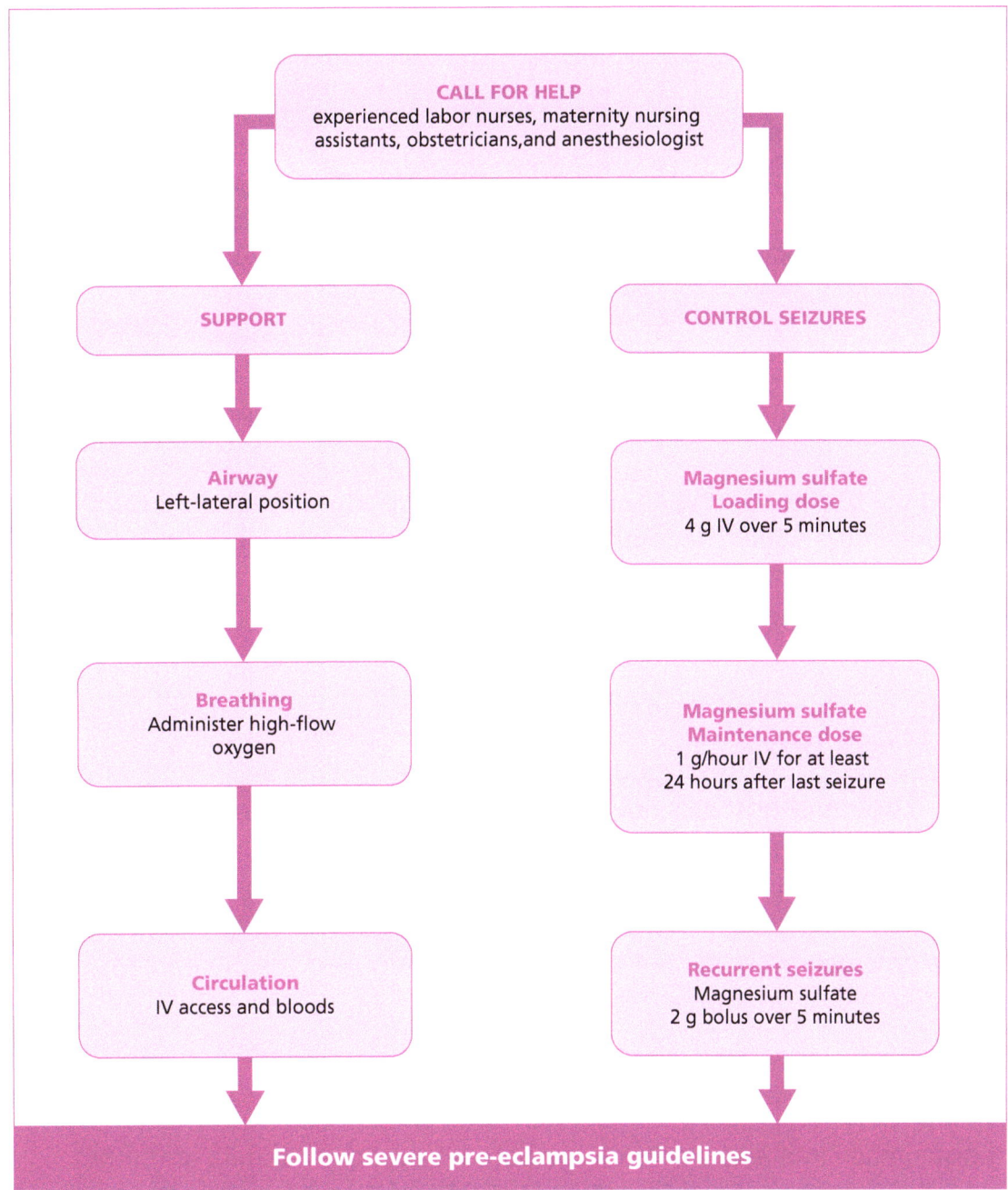

Figure 6.1 Outline for the initial management of eclampsia

Support: airway, breathing, circulation

Remember that most seizures are self-limited and it is important that those who are involved with the patient's care remain calm. As your first priority, monitor and maintain the maternal airway, breathing, and circulation. Move the mother to the left-lateral position and protect her from injury. Provide high-flow oxygen by facemask with a reservoir bag. Do not attempt to restrain her

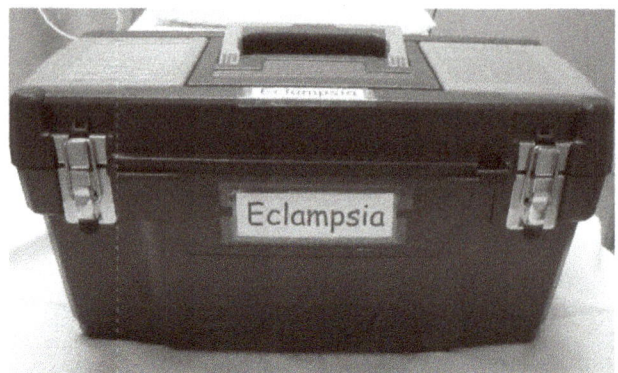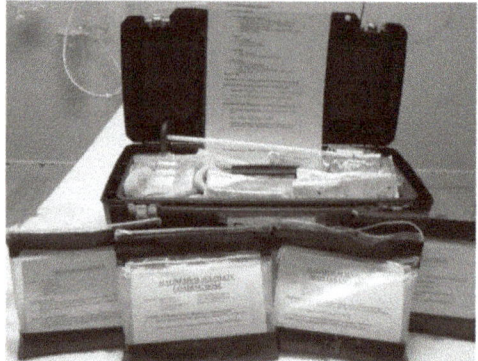

Figure 6.2 Eclampsia box with laminated treatment algorithm attached and showing contents

during the seizure. During a seizure, it is also important to refrain from placing anything in the patient's mouth for the purpose of maintaining airway patency as this could lead to self-injury in addition to causing more harm than benefit to the patient. However, be sure the woman remains in the left-lateral position with an open airway immediately following the eclamptic seizure.

Eclampsia box

Many if not most hospitals now keep all medications required for eclampsia in an automated pharmacy dispensing unit with the magnesium sulfate premixed and ready to administer. If this is not the case at your hospital, it is wise to prepare an emergency box containing a laminated treatment protocol as well as the emergency equipment and medication required for the immediate management of eclampsia (Figure 6.2).

Control of seizures

If not already in place, insert a large-bore intravenous cannula and if not recently performed, obtain samples for CBC, urea and electrolytes, liver function tests, clotting and a blood type and hold. Begin an infusion of magnesium sulfate – 4 g loading dose followed by 1 g per hour.

> **Do not use diazepam, phenytoin, or lytic cocktail as an alternative to magnesium sulfate in women with eclampsia.**

The results of the Collaborative Eclampsia Trial demonstrated that women treated with magnesium sulfate have fewer recurrent seizures compared with women treated with diazepam or phenytoin.[9] Magnesium sulfate appears to act primarily to reduce cerebral vasospasm.[10] The intravenous route is preferred as intramuscular injections are painful and complicated by local abscess formation in 0.5% of cases. The MAGPIE Trial demonstrated that magnesium sulfate can also prevent primary eclampsia (although the number of women needing treatment to prevent one having an eclamptic seizure is high, particularly in the developed world).[11]

Magnesium sulfate emergency regimen

Loading dose: 4 g magnesium sulfate over 5 minutes

- If not available as a redi-mix, draw up 8 ml of 50% magnesium sulfate solution (4 g) followed by 12 ml of 0.9% normal saline into a 20 ml syringe. This will give a total volume of 20 ml
- Give manually as an intravenous bolus over 5 minutes

Maintenance dose: 1 g/hour

- If not available as a redi-mix, draw up 40 ml of magnesium sulfate solution (5 g per 10 ml) and inject into a liter of crystalloid
- Infuse at 50 ml/hour (approximately 1 g per hour)
- Continue infusion until a postpartum diuresis occurs (>200 ml per hour for at least 2 hours) or for 24 hours following delivery

Recurrent seizures while on magnesium sulfate

- Seek immediate experienced help
- Give an additional 2 g bolus of magnesium sulfate
- If possible, take blood for magnesium levels prior to giving the bolus dose

The maternal condition must be stabilized prior to making plans for delivery (if antenatal).

Recurrent seizures may require treatment with diazepam or thiopental/propofol (if an anesthesiologist is present). In that instance, consider other causes of seizures, such as intracranial hemorrhage, epilepsy, a space-occupying cerebral lesion or a cerebral vein thrombosis, and obtain emergent imaging (CT, MRI) as appropriate.

Magnesium sulfate is excreted in urine by the kidneys and pre-eclampsia alters excretion. Magnesium toxicity is unlikely with the 1 g per hour regimen, and if

> **Box 6.4 Magnesium sulfate emergency protocol**
>
> CARDIOPULMONARY ARREST ON MAGNESIUM SULFATE
>
> - Stop magnesium sulfate infusion
> - Start basic life support
> - Give 1 g calcium gluconate IV (10 ml of 10% solution)
> - Intubate early and ventilate until respiration resumes

the woman has a normal urine output, routine measurement of magnesium levels is unnecessary. However, if the woman is oliguric (less than 100 ml urine over 4 hours) or has known renal impairment, magnesium levels are more likely to become elevated over time, and it may be advisable to administer the loading dose only. The therapeutic range for magnesium sulfate treatment is 2–4 mmol/l (4.8–8.4 mg/dl).If the woman develops oliguria while receiving the maintenance dose of the magnesium sulfate, it should be stopped or decreased, and blood taken to measure the serum magnesium level.

At toxic levels, there is a loss of deep tendon reflexes followed by respiratory depression, respiratory arrest, and, ultimately, cardiac arrest. If maternal collapse occurs, follow the emergency protocol in Box 6.4. If toxicity is suspected, immediately stop the magnesium sulfate infusion and take blood for magnesium levels.

Documentation

All personnel present at the emergency and all actions and treatment administered should be recorded as contemporaneously as possible. Figure 6.3 gives an example of an eclampsia documentation template that may be used.

Severe pre-eclampsia management guidelines

Severe pre-eclampsia has been defined as:[4]

- Severe hypertension (BP ≥160/110 mmHg) and proteinuria (either a urinary protein:creatinine ratio >30 mg/mmol or a 24-hour urine collection with >300 mg protein)

PROMPT
Making Childbirth Safer, Together

ECLAMPSIA TEMPLATE

DATE .... TIME OF SEIZURE: .... DURATION OF SEIZURE: ....

PERSONS PRESENT AT ONSET OF SEIZURE ....

....

EMERGENCY ALARM ACTIVATED   YES / NO   TIME ....

If emergency alarm not activated, please give reason ....

	NAME	ALREADY PRESENT (✓)	TIME INFORMED	TIME ARRIVED
EXPERIENCED OBSTETRICIAN				
NURSING COORDINATOR				
ANESTHESIOLOGIST				
TRAINEES				
TECHNICIANS				
OTHER PERSONS ASSISTING				

TREATMENT

LEFT LATERAL POSITION   YES / NO   TIME .... If no, other position ....

HIGH FLOW O_2 YES / NO   TIME .... If no, give reason ....

IV ACCESS   YES / NO   TIME .... If no, give reason ....

BLOODS – TYPE + HOLD   YES / NO   TIME .... If no, give reason ....
(CBC, CLOTTING, ELECTROLYTES,
URIC ACID, LFT's)

MAGNESIUM SULFATE INFUSION (see laminated regimen for dosages)	TIME INITIATED
LOADING DOSE	
MAINTENANCE DOSE	

INITIAL POST SEIZURE VITAL SIGNS   TIME.................

RESP RATE........... PULSE RATE .... BP...........mm/Hg O_2 sats ....% TEMP.................°C

URINARY CATHETER INSERTED   YES / NO   TIME............. If no, give reason..

(Begin Critical Care Charting)

HYPERTENSIVE TREATMENT ADMINISTERED   YES / NO   TIME ....
if yes, please document medication given and dosage ....

....

Figure 6.3 Example of eclampsia documentation proforma

or

- Mild or moderate hypertension (BP 140/90–159/109 mmHg) and proteinuria with at least one of the following:
  - ☐ severe headache
  - ☐ problems with vision such as blurring or flashing
  - ☐ severe pain just below ribs or vomiting
  - ☐ papilledema
  - ☐ signs of clonus ($\geq$3 beats)
  - ☐ liver tenderness
  - ☐ platelet count below 100,000 platelets/microliter
  - ☐ abnormal liver enzymes (ALT or AST rises to >70 i.u./l)
  - ☐ HELLP syndrome.

Note: clinical discretion should be used to include women who present with atypical symptoms.[12]

Details of the management principles are outlined in Figure 6.4. These principles are discussed in more detail in the following section.

Management principles

The management of severe pre-eclampsia and eclampsia requires the initiation of complex treatment plans.[13]

1. Stabilize

Effective and timely antihypertensive treatment is vital.[3,4]

Control of hypertension

A major failing in the critical care deaths of women with eclampsia and severe pre-eclampsia is inadequate treatment of systolic hypertension, resulting in intracranial hemorrhage before therapy has either been given or had the opportunity to work.[3] The exact mechanisms that link hypertension with intracranial hemorrhage are still unclear, but systolic hypertension poses the greatest risk. In addition, mean arterial pressure measurements may not always impart the real threat of a very high systolic blood pressure. Based on the evidence available, a systolic pressure of 160 mmHg or more requires urgent and effective antihypertensive treatment.[5] *But because pre-eclampsia can worsen rapidly, and the threat of intracranial*

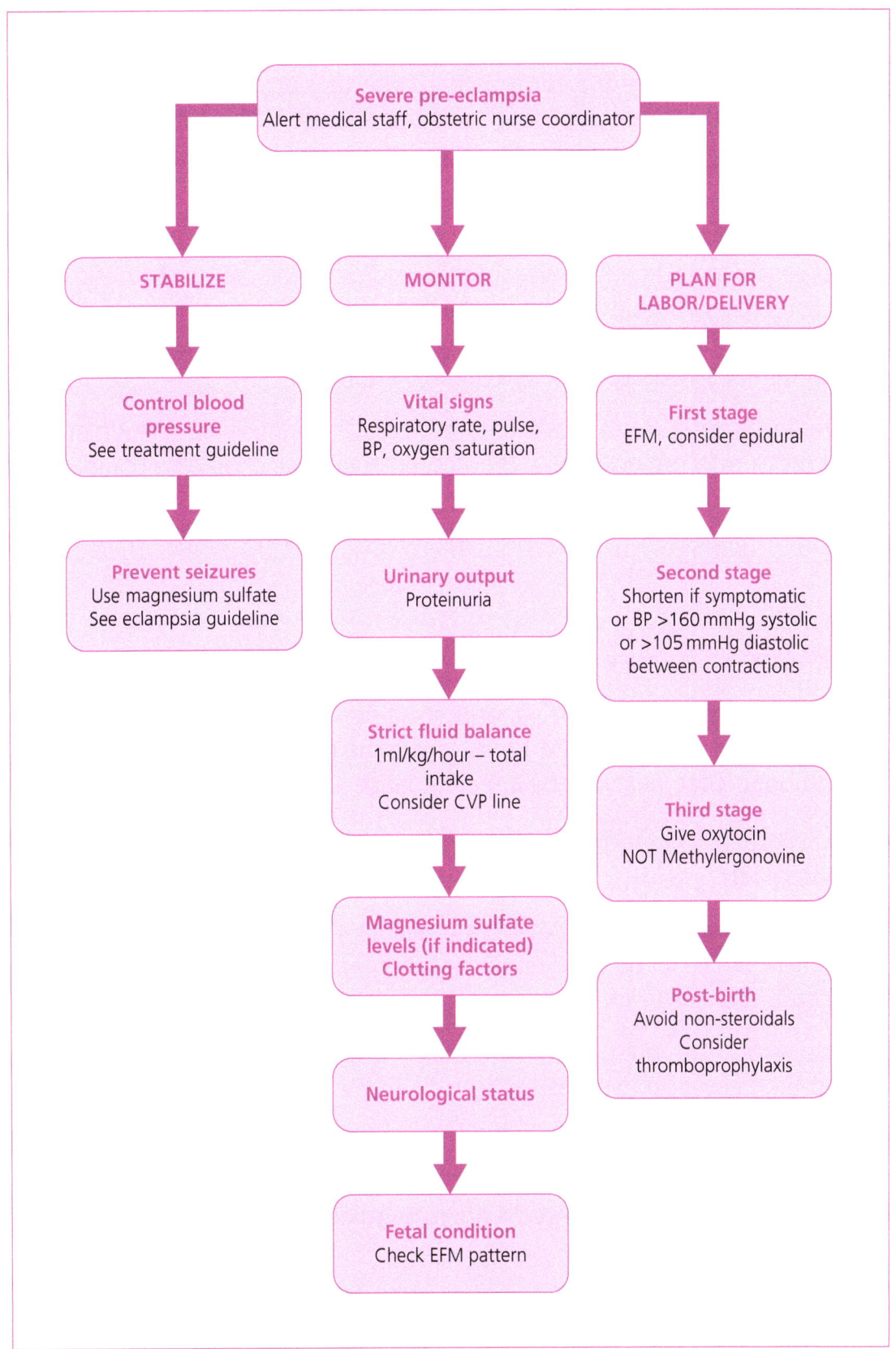

Figure 6.4 Suggested outline of the management of severe pre-eclampsia

hemorrhage escalates above 160 mmHg, it is wise to initiate antihypertensive agents when the systolic blood pressure exceeds 150 mmHg (see Figure 6.5 for a severe hypertension treatment flow chart). As a result of these two reports[3,5] and the release of the NICE report on treatment of hypertension, deaths from intracranial hemorrhage have declined.[14]

Any prescribed antihypertensive medication should be continued in labor and at cesarean section (usually labetalol and/or nifedipine). Anesthesiologists and obstetricians should also be aware of the hypertensive effects of laryngoscopy and intubation when administering a general anesthetic and control the maternal hypertension prior to intubation.[3]

Automated blood pressure recording devices can seriously underestimate blood pressure in pre-eclampsia. Blood pressure values should be compared at the beginning of treatment with those obtained by a manual device with an appropriately sized cuff.[11] Consideration should be given to the use of an arterial line for difficult cases.

Prevention of seizures

Consider giving intravenous magnesium sulfate to women with pre-eclampsia if delivery is planned within 24 hours as per the eclampsia regimen; that is, a loading bolus dose followed by a maintenance infusion.

2. Monitor

The maternal condition can deteriorate rapidly. Close observation and assessment are required and should be recorded on an obstetric critical care chart.

- Respiratory rate, pulse and blood pressure: every 15 minutes until stabile, and then every 30 minutes.
- Hourly urine output: Foley catheter with urometer.
- Hourly oxygen saturations.
- Routine blood samples every 24 hours or as indicated: CBC, clotting screen, BUN, electrolytes, LFTs.

Additional observations and investigation for mothers receiving magnesium sulfate:

- continuously monitor oxygen saturation
- hourly respiratory rate

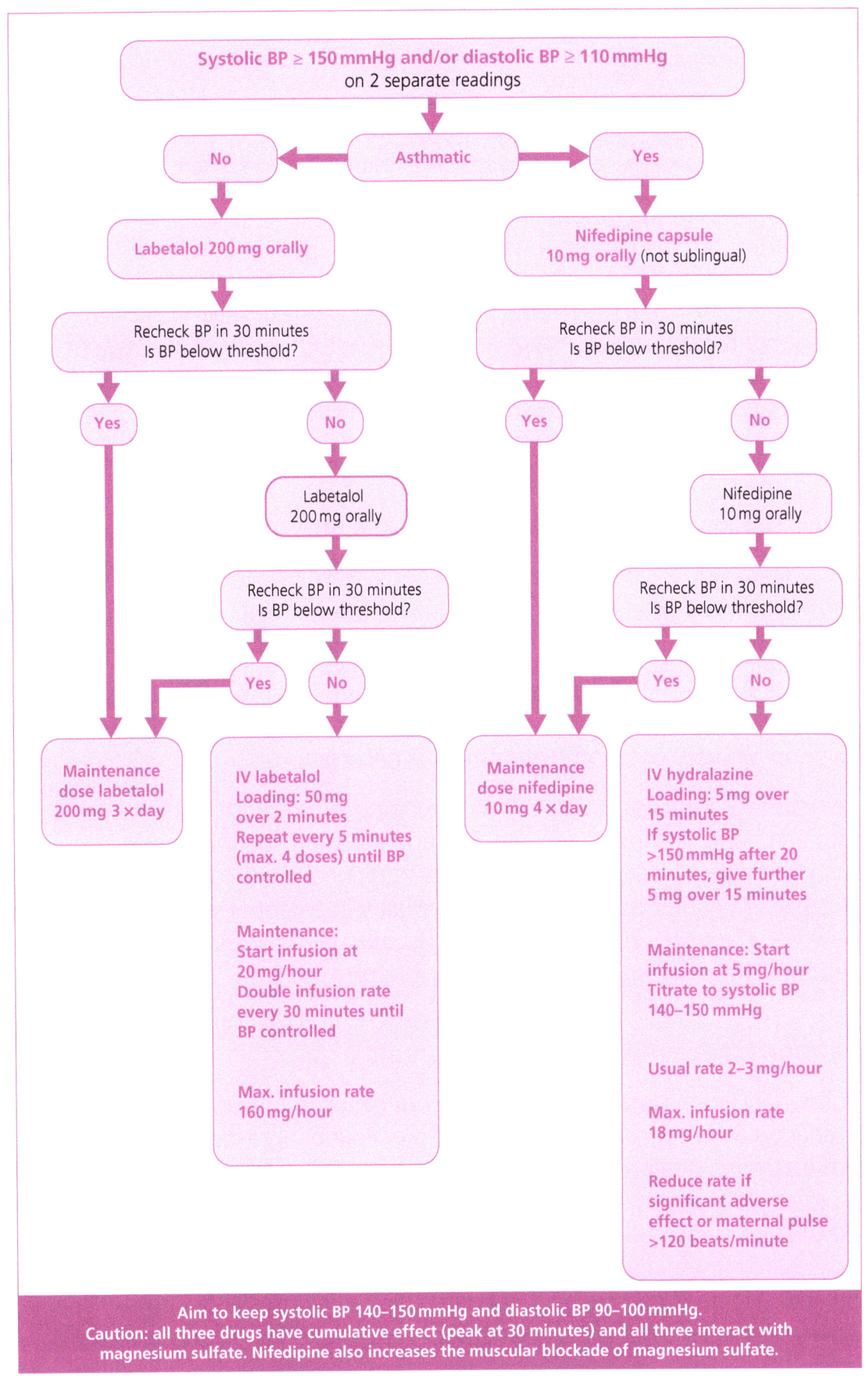

Figure 6.5 Suggested treatment guidelines for severe hypertension

- if oliguric (less than 100 ml urine in 4 hours), magnesium levels every 4 hours
- hourly deep tendon reflexes if oliguric
- if loss of reflexes, stop infusion and check magnesium levels:
  - □ if level less than 4 mmol/l (<8.4 mg/dl) or reflexes return, resume the infusion at 0.5 g/hour.

Strict fluid balance

Close monitoring of fluid intake and urinary output is essential. Previous postmortem reviews have highlighted the risk of fluid overload causing pulmonary edema in women with severe pre-eclampsia.

The maximum fluid intake (a combination of intravenous and oral intake) should be 1 ml/kg/hour (often approximated to 80 ml/hour). Beware of dilute drug administration and of excessive oxytocin, which may inhibit urinary output.

All women with severe pre-eclampsia should have an indwelling urinary catheter, with a urometer for hourly urine measurement. All fluid input and output should be clearly documented on an obstetric critical care chart.

The goal is to "run her dry," as women die from fluid overload but rarely from renal failure. The intravenous fluid of choice for most cases will be Ringer's solution or D_5NS or blood replacement if necessary.

Persistent oliguria (less than 100 ml of urine over 4 hours) requires careful management, as shown in Figure 6.6, and a central line may aid fluid management, especially when there are additional complications such as a postpartum hemorrhage. The aim is to maintain a central venous pressure between 0 mmHg and 5 mmHg. Exercise caution with fluid treatment if the central venous pressure is greater than 5 mmHg.

Pulmonary edema

Pulmonary edema is defined as fluid accumulation in the lungs that impairs gas exchange and may cause respiratory failure. Pulmonary edema in women with pre-eclampsia reflects hypoalbuminemia, increased capillary permeability, and a high hydrostatic pressure (hypertension). Fortunately, pulmonary edema is now a rare complication of pre-eclampsia as it has been recognized that it is essential to restrict fluids ("run the patient dry") and maintain an accurate fluid balance. Figure 6.7 shows an X-ray of the typical features of pulmonary edema; however, clinical signs are usually sufficient to make the diagnosis (Box 6.5).

The immediate management of pulmonary edema is shown in Figure 6.8.

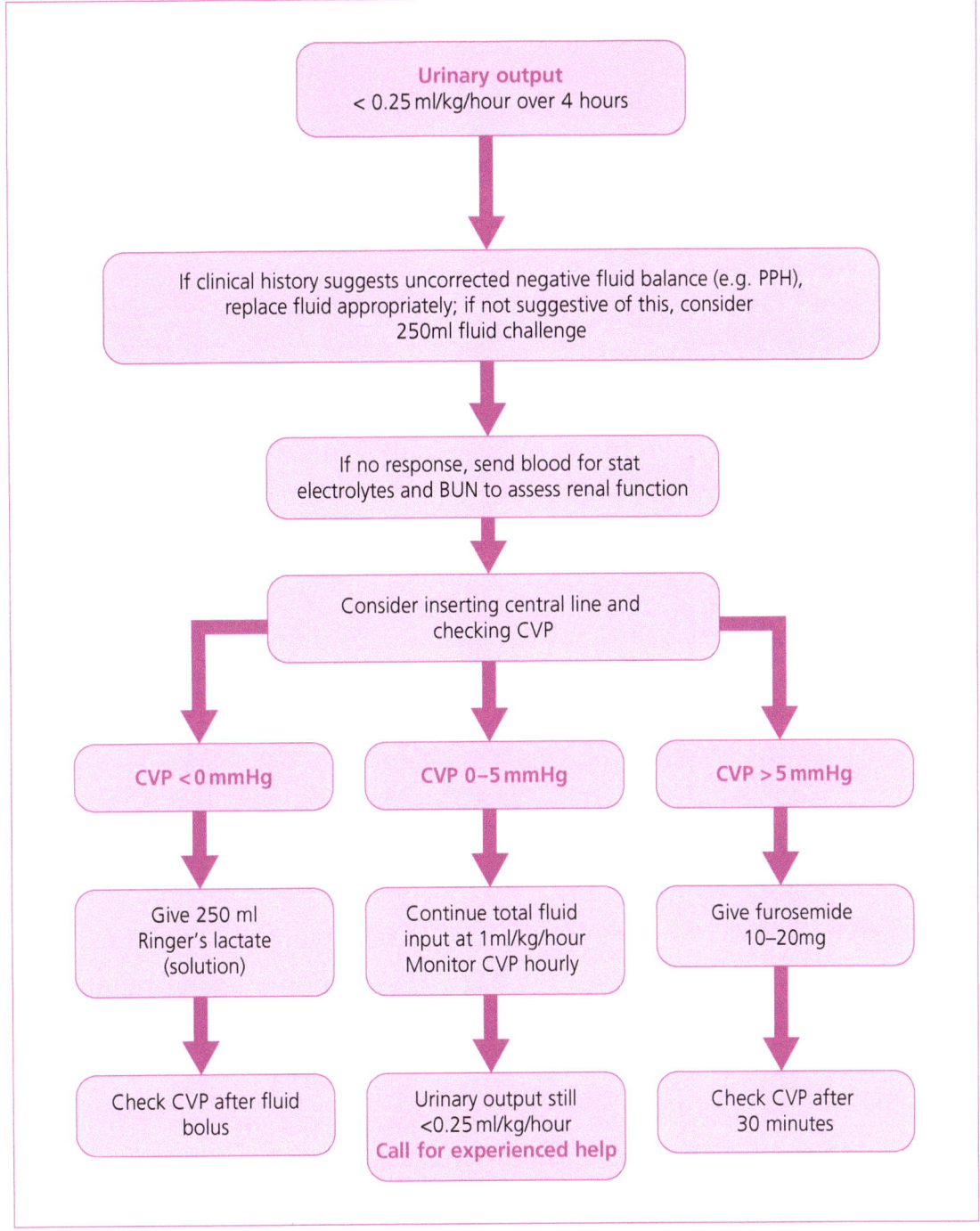

Figure 6.6 Fluid balance in the mother with oliguric pre-eclampsia

Clotting abnormalities

The clinical syndrome of disseminated intravascular coagulation (DIC) is a potential complication of severe pre-eclampsia. Check the activated partial thromboplastin time (aPTT), prothrombin time, and fibrinogen if the platelet counts are below 100,000 platelets per microliter. Observe for clinical evidence of undue bleeding/bruises. If any of the investigations are abnormal, consider

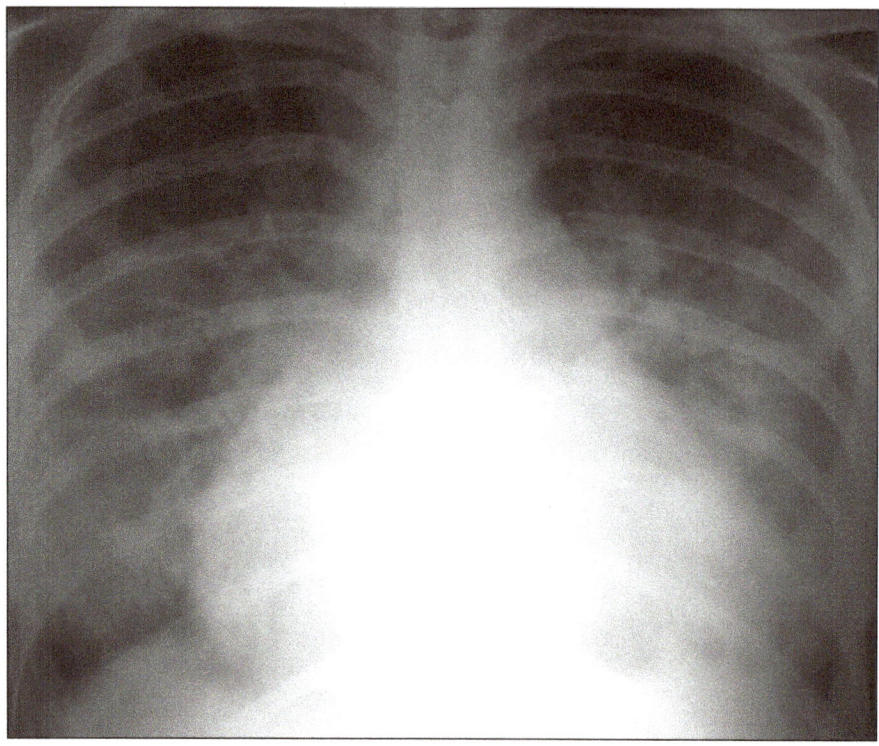

Figure 6.7 Chest X-ray showing the features of pulmonary edema

---

Box 6.5 Clinical signs and symptoms of pulmonary edema

Symptoms of pulmonary edema	Signs of pulmonary edema
Shortness of breath	Tachypnea
Unable to lie flat	Crepitations at lung bases
	Decreasing oxygen saturations
	Positive fluid balance
	Tachycardia
	Frothy sputum

---

treatment with platelets and fresh frozen plasma (FFP) and consultation with a hematologist (more information can be found in Module 2).

3. Plan for labor/delivery

Make plans for delivery in women with severe pre-eclampsia once the mother's condition is stable. The choice of cesarean section or induction of labor should be individualized. During the 1st stage of labor, the continuous attendance of an experienced labor nurse is required.

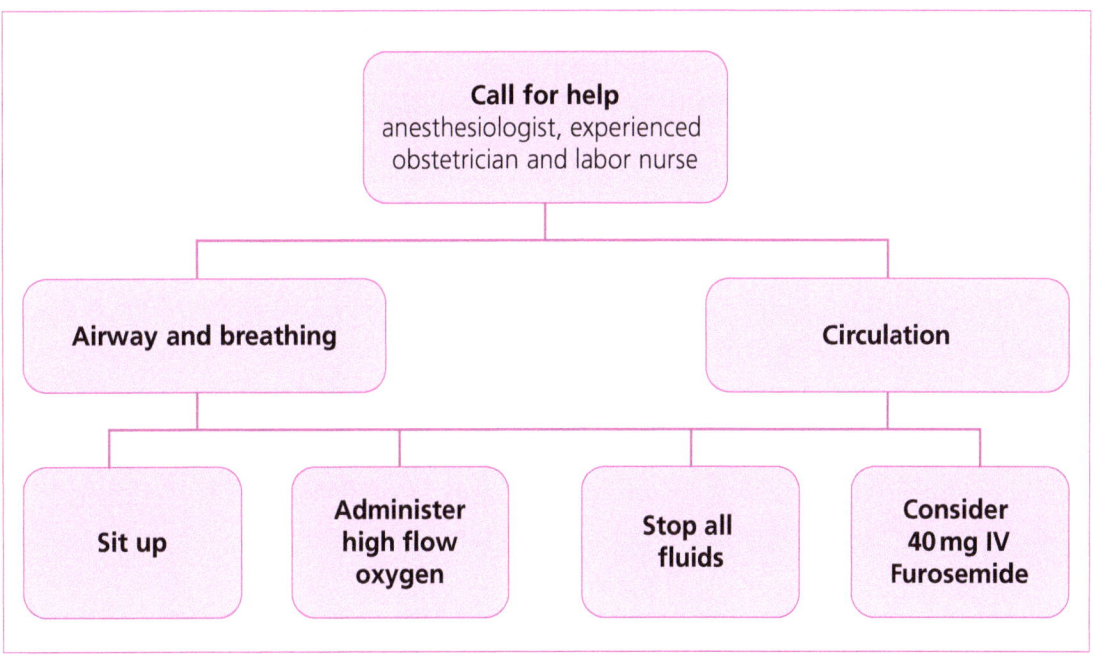

Figure 6.8 Immediate management of pulmonary edema

- Use continuous EFM: there is an increased risk of fetal hypoxia and placental abruption.

- Consider the use of epidural anesthesia (pain tends to increase blood pressure). Do not preload women with IV fluids prior to epidural or spinal.[4]

- During labor, measure the BP every 15 minutes in women with severe hypertension or hourly in women with mild or moderate hypertension.

It is safe for the mother to have a normal 2nd stage of labor provided that she does not have a severe headache or visual disturbances and that her blood pressure is within acceptable limits.

Consider operative vaginal birth if:

- the mother complains of severe headache or visual disturbances
- the blood pressure is uncontrolled (greater than 160 mmHg systolic or 105 mmHg diastolic, between contractions) *despite* treatment.

The 3rd stage of labor should be actively managed to reduce the risk of postpartum hemorrhage (oxytocin and misoprostil). Methergine is relatively contraindicated in women with pre-eclampsia or eclampsia as it exacerbates hypertension.

Post-birth care

The mother will require continuous care after delivery. This may be for several hours or several days, depending on when the expected postpartum diuresis occurs and control of the hypertension is achieved. Remember that some eclamptic seizures occur in the postnatal period, and pre-eclampsia can worsen several days after birth if the maternal diuresis has not occurred. If symptoms arise, monitor and investigate. Women may require transfer back to the labor floor for clinical monitoring.

Ensure adequate analgesia but non-steroidal anti-inflammatory drugs such as ibuprofen or indomethacin should be avoided as they can precipitate renal failure and exacerbate hypertension.

Strongly consider thromboprophylaxis, as severe pre-eclampsia is a risk factor for thromboembolism. Apply anti-thromboembolic stockings as soon as possible. Begin low-molecular-weight heparin after delivery if the mother's platelet count is greater than 100×10^9/liter.

Transfer to intensive therapy unit or high-dependency care

Women should be managed in the appropriate setting,[5] which should reflect your hospital's infrastructure (Table 6.1). Labor units should have documented

Table 6.1 Treatment settings

Setting	Indication
Level 3 care: ICU	Severe pre-eclampsia requiring ventilation
Level 2 care: high-dependency care perhaps in the labor unit	Step down from Level 3 or severe pre-eclampsia with either: ■ eclampsia ■ HELLP syndrome ■ hemorrhage ■ hyperkalemia ■ severe oliguria ■ coagulopathy support ■ IV antihypertensive treatment ■ initial stabilization of severe hypertension ■ evidence of cardiac failure ■ abnormal neurology

Table 6.1 (*cont.*)

Setting	Indication
Level 1 care: postpartum with the assistance of a critical care team	■ Pre-eclampsia with mild or moderate hypertension input ■ Continuing conservative antenatal management of severe preterm hypertension ■ Step-down treatment after the birth

procedures for the transfer of a mother to an ICU (recognizes some labor units have ICU capabilities that would obviate the need for transfer).[5]

References

1. Khan KS, Wojdyla D, Say L, Gülmezoglu AM, Van Look PF. WHO analysis of causes of maternal death: a systematic review. *Lancet* 2006; 367: 1066–74.

2. Creanga AA, Berg CJ, Syverson C, Seed K, Bruce FC, Callaghan WM. Pregnancy-related mortality in the United States, 2006–2010. *Obstet Gynecol* 2015; 125(1): 5–12.

3. Centre for Maternal and Child Enquiries. Saving Mothers' Lives: reviewing maternal deaths to make motherhood safer: 2006–2008. The Eighth Report on Confidential Enquiries into Maternal Deaths in the United Kingdom. *BJOG* 2011; 118 (Suppl 1): 1–203.

4. Lewis G (ed.) *The Confidential Enquiry into Maternal and Child Health (CEMACH). Saving Mothers' Lives: Reviewing Maternal Deaths to Make Motherhood Safer 2003–2005. The Seventh Report on Confidential Enquiries into Maternal Deaths in the United Kingdom.* London: CEMACH; 2007.

5. National Collaborating Centre for Women's and Children's Health. *Hypertension in Pregnancy: the Management of Hypertensive Disorders during Pregnancy. NICE Clinical Guideline.* London: Royal College of Obstetricians and Gynaecologists; 2011.

6. Ananth CV, Keyes KM, Wapner RJ. Pre-eclampsia rates in the United States, 1980–2010: age-period-cohort analysis. *BMJ* 2013; Nov 7; 347: f6564. doi: 10.1136/bmj.f6564.

7. Knight M, UKOSS. Eclampsia in the United Kingdom 2005. *BJOG* 2007; 114: 1072–8.

8. Wallis AB, Saftlas AF, Hsia J, Atrash HK. Secular trends in the rates of preeclampsia, eclampsia, and gestational hypertension, United States, 1987–2004. *Am J Hyperten* 2008: 21: 521–6.

9. Which anticonvulsant for women with eclampsia? Evidence from the Collaborative Eclampsia Trial. *Lancet* 1995; 345: 1455–63.

10. Naidu S, Payne AJ, Moodley J, Hoffmann M, Gouws E. Randomised study assessing the effect of phenytoin and magnesium sulfate on maternal cerebral circulation in eclampsia using transcranial Doppler ultrasound. *Br J Obstet Gynaecol* 1996; 103: 111–16.

11. Altman D, Carroli G, Duley L, Farrell B, Moodley J, Neilson J, et al. Magpie Trial Collaboration Group. Do women with pre-eclampsia, and their babies, benefit from magnesium sulfate? The Magpie Trial: a randomised placebo-controlled trial. *Lancet* 2002; 359: 1877–90.

12. Lewis G (ed.) *The Confidential Enquiry into Maternal and Child Health (CEMACH).Why Mothers Die 2000–2002. The Sixth Report on Confidential Enquiries into Maternal Deaths in the United Kingdom*. London: RCOG Press; 2004.

13. Royal College of Obstetricians and Gynaecologists. *The Management of Severe Pre-eclampsia/ eclampsia. Green-top Guideline No. 10A*. London: RCOG; 2006.

14. Knight M, Kenyon S, Brocklehurst P, Neilson J, Shakespeare J, Kurinczuk JJ (eds) on behalf of MBRRACEUK. *Saving Lives, Improving Mothers' Care: Lessons Learned to Inform Future Maternity Care from the UK and Ireland Confidential Enquiries into Maternal Deaths and Morbidity 2009–12*. Oxford: National Perinatal Epidemiology Unit, University of Oxford; 2014.

Module 7
Maternal sepsis

Key learning points

- Recognize severe maternal sepsis.
- Use serum lactate to triage sepsis severity.
- Understand the steps for the emergency management of septic shock.
- Recognize the need for early intravenous antibiotics and fluids.
- Importance of adopting and using modified obstetric early warning score (MOEWS) charts.
- Recognize the importance of early involvement of experienced, multi-professional clinicians.
- Recall the potential complications of severe sepsis.
- Encourage influenza vaccination for all pregnant women unless clearly contraindicated.

Common difficulties observed in training drills

- Not stating the problem.
- Failing to measure the patient's respiratory rate.
- Not plotting clinical observations on a MOEWS chart.
- Failing to recognize clinical features of sepsis.
- Delaying antibiotic administration.
- Failing to treat sepsis with a fluid bolus.
- Failing to obtain microbiology cultures and serum lactate.
- Failing to summon appropriate experienced support early.

Introduction

Obstetricians and midwives of the past were very aware of sepsis and its consequences. Before the introduction of antibiotics in the 1940s, genital tract sepsis was a leading cause of maternal death, accounting for over one-third of direct deaths occurring in pregnancy and childbirth. Since the introduction of antibiotics the number of maternal deaths attributable to sepsis has fallen dramatically. As a result many doctors and midwives have never managed severe maternal sepsis.

There has recently been a growing concern, both in the United States and the UK, that the percentage of maternal deaths attributable to sepsis has increased.[1] From 2006 to 2010, 166 women died of sepsis or chorioamnionitis in the United States. Alarmingly, another 242 women died of "other" infectious complications. In total, infection was the cause of 456 maternal deaths, the 3rd highest cause (Table 7.1). The more detailed Confidential Enquiries in the UK observed during a similar time period that sepsis was the leading cause of direct maternal deaths, particularly those associated with group A streptococcal (GAS) infection (Table 7.2).[2] The majority of these deaths occurred postpartum, and more than 50% followed cesarean delivery. However, seven women died from sepsis after vaginal birth, highlighting that even a healthy woman with a normal pregnancy and delivery can become rapidly ill and die.

The news is not all bad. The recent MBBRACE report noted an encouraging decline in genital tract sepsis since 2008, suggesting the recent emphasis on early recognition, the Surviving Sepsis campaign and Sepsis

Table 7.1 Number and proportion of maternal deaths from infection in the United States

Cause of death	Live birth	Stillbirth	Ectopic	Abortion	Undelivered	Unknown	Total
Infection	251 (12.5%)	35 (22.2%)	1 (1.0%)	42 (46.7%)	80 (12.1%)	47 (13.8%)	456 (13.6%)
Chorioamnionitis	5	6	0	3	6	2	22 (0.7%)
Genital tract	34	2	0	6	2	4	48 (1.4%)
Sepsis	63	19	0	30	22	10	144 (4.3%)
Other or unspecified	149	8	1	3	50	31	242 (7.2%)

Table 7.2 Number and proportion of maternal deaths from sepsis in the UK

	1952–54	1985–87	2000–02	2003–05	2006–08
Rate/100,000 maternities	7.8	0.40	0.65	0.85	1.13
Number (all organisms)	–	9	13	21	29
Number (GAS)	–	–	3	8	13

Six (discussed subsequently), and the encouragement of influenza vaccination does indeed work.[3]

Worldwide, sepsis remains a very important cause of maternal death: in one year alone (2005), over 80,000 women across the world died from pregnancy-related sepsis.[4]

What is sepsis?

Sepsis is the body's response following invasion by microorganisms, usually bacteria. The infection may be limited to a particular body region (e.g., chorioamnionitis) or may be widespread in the bloodstream, resulting in septicemia. Sepsis is a medical emergency because it can result in an interruption of the supply of oxygen and nutrients to the tissues, including the vital organs such as the brain, heart, liver, kidneys, lungs, and intestines, resulting in acidosis, organ failure, and death.

Prevention of sepsis

The importance of hand washing, hygiene, and antiseptics is well established in obstetric care. In the mid-19th century, Semmelweis observed a marked increase in the maternal mortality rates of women under the care of doctors compared to those of midwives in Vienna. He also noted that doctors coming straight from the autopsy room to the delivery room had a disagreeable smell on their hands despite washing with plain soap and water. He hypothesized that puerperal fever was caused by particles transmitted via the hands of the doctors. Semmelweis ordered a mandatory hand-washing policy for doctors, requiring them to use a chlorinated solution before they examined women in labor. This intervention produced a dramatic fall in maternal mortality.[5]

Other techniques to reduce maternal sepsis include routine influenza vaccination of pregnant women, barrier nursing, the use of antibiotic prophylaxis for preterm and prolonged rupture of membranes, and the use of perioperative antibiotics for cesarean births, manual removal of the placenta, and anal sphincter tear repair.

Recognition of sepsis

The onset of life-threatening sepsis in pregnancy or the puerperium can range from insidious to extremely rapid clinical deterioration, particularly when it is caused by streptococcal infection. In many of the sepsis-related maternal deaths reviewed by the Confidential Enquiries, women had a short duration of illness and in some cases were moribund by the time they were admitted to the hospital.

It is therefore essential that all staff, including labor suite nurses, community midwives, emergency department staff, and family medicine and pediatric practitioners, are aware of the signs and symptoms of sepsis. "Think sepsis" at an early stage when presented with an ill pregnant or recently pregnant woman, take appropriate observations, and act on them.[3] The severity of illness in women presenting with signs and symptoms of sepsis is often unrecognized or underestimated, resulting in delays in hospitalization, delays in administration of appropriate antibiotic treatment, and late involvement of experienced medical staff.[6] It is equally important that women themselves be informed of the risks, signs, and symptoms of genital tract infection and the need for them to seek early advice if they are concerned.[2]

Signs and symptoms

Women with genital tract sepsis may present with abdominal pain, diarrhea, and vomiting. Some, but not all, will have a fever. It may be difficult to differentiate such symptoms from gastroenteritis, and as a result, all pregnant or postpartum women presenting with such symptoms should be carefully examined. Women may also present antenatally with a foul smelling vaginal discharge, or with increased and/or foul smelling lochia in the puerperium. Antenatally, the combination of abdominal pain and an abnormal or absent fetal heart rate may signify sepsis rather than placental abruption.

Many of the deaths are preceded by a sore throat or other upper respiratory tract infections.[2] Many of the women who die from GAS either work with, or have, young children. The typical rash of streptococcus A (Figure 7.1) develops over 12 to 48 hours, first appearing as erythematous (red) patches on the chest and axillae, which spread to the trunk and extremities. Typically, the rash consists of scarlet patches over generalized redness (a patchy sunburnt

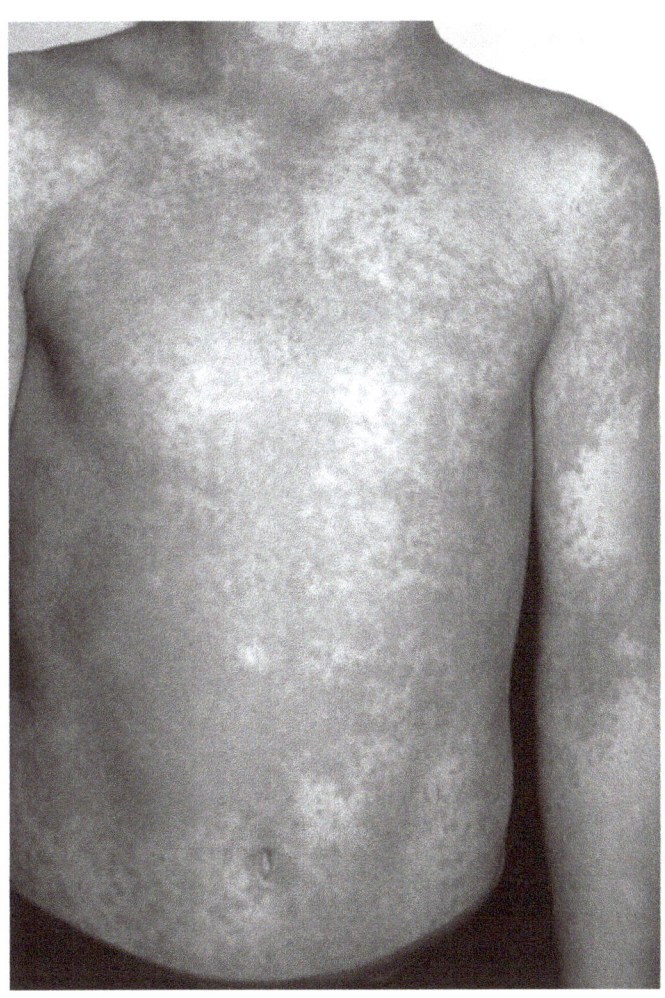

Figure 7.1 Streptococcus A rash

appearance). This rash will momentarily disappear with pressure, unlike the petechial rash typical of meningococcal septicemia.

Women with severe sepsis can seem deceptively well. They may maintain their blood pressure and conceal serious illness for a prolonged period of time before suddenly decompensating. It is vital that basic vital signs (heart rate, respiratory rate, blood pressure, temperature, and, if available, oxygen saturations) are taken from every woman who presents with any of the symptoms in Box 7.1, or who simply "just doesn't feel well." The use of modified obstetric early warning score (MOEWS) charts to record physical observations is recommended, and should help in the early detection of women with sepsis.

Risk factors

Risk factors for sepsis are listed in Box 7.2 and potential causes of sepsis are listed in Box 7.3. However, many women who present with sepsis have no risk

Box 7.1 Signs and symptoms of genital tract sepsis

Symptoms	Signs
Fever	Rash (scarlet patches over generalized redness or petechiae)
Diarrhea	Tachycardia (heart rate >100 bpm)
Vomiting	Tachypnea/raised respiratory rate (respiratory rate >24)
Abdominal pain	Fever (>38°C) or hypothermia (<35°C)
	Hypotension (systolic blood pressure <80 mmHg)
Sore throat	Low oxygen saturations (<95% on air)
	Poor peripheral perfusion (capillary refill >2 seconds)
Upper respiratory tract infection	Pallor
Vaginal discharge	Clamminess
Wound infection	Confusion
	Mottled skin
	Low urine output (<0.5 ml/kg/hour)

Box 7.2 Risk factors for maternal sepsis

- Retained products of conception (following miscarriage, pregnancy termination, or delivery)
- Cesarean delivery (emergency cesarean has a greater risk than an elective or planned cesarean)
- Prolonged ruptured membranes
- Premature labor
- Water birth
- Wound hematoma
- After an invasive intrauterine procedure (e.g., amniocentesis, chorionic villus sampling)
- Cervical cerclage
- Obesity
- Impaired immunity (e.g., immunosuppressants, high-dose steroids, HIV infection)
- Diabetes mellitus
- Working with, or having, young children

Box 7.3 Potential pregnancy- and non-pregnancy-related causes of maternal sepsis

Pregnancy related	Non-pregnancy related
Chorioamnionitis (after retained products of conception, prolonged ruptured membranes, cesarean delivery, invasive procedures)	Appendicitis (may present atypically in pregnancy)
	Pyelonephritis (more common in pregnancy)
	Cholecystitis
Postoperative (cesarean delivery, cervical cerclage, hematoma, amniocentesis)	Bowel perforation (more common with inflammatory bowel disease)
Breast abscesses	Meningitis
	Pneumonia
	Cellulitis

factors. In a postpartum woman with possible sepsis, a history consistent with incomplete delivery of the placenta or fetal membranes should be sought, and the woman examined for the presence of uterine tenderness or enlargement.

Management

The Surviving Sepsis Campaign is a global initiative aimed at reducing mortality from sepsis by building awareness, improving diagnosis, increasing the use of appropriate treatment, educating healthcare professionals, and developing guidelines for care. More information about the Surviving Sepsis Campaign can be found at www.survivingsepsis.org.[7]

Maternal sepsis can be challenging to manage, but better training, a structured approach, earlier recognition, and good care in both community and hospital settings will save lives. The optimal management of severe maternal sepsis requires the rapid initiation of several overlapping actions. The exact sequence is dictated by the needs of the individual mother and the resources available but requires timely recognition, rapid administration of appropriate intravenous antibiotics, and consultation with experienced physicians. An outline for the initial management of sepsis is shown in Figure 7.2. Management is described in more detail in the next section.

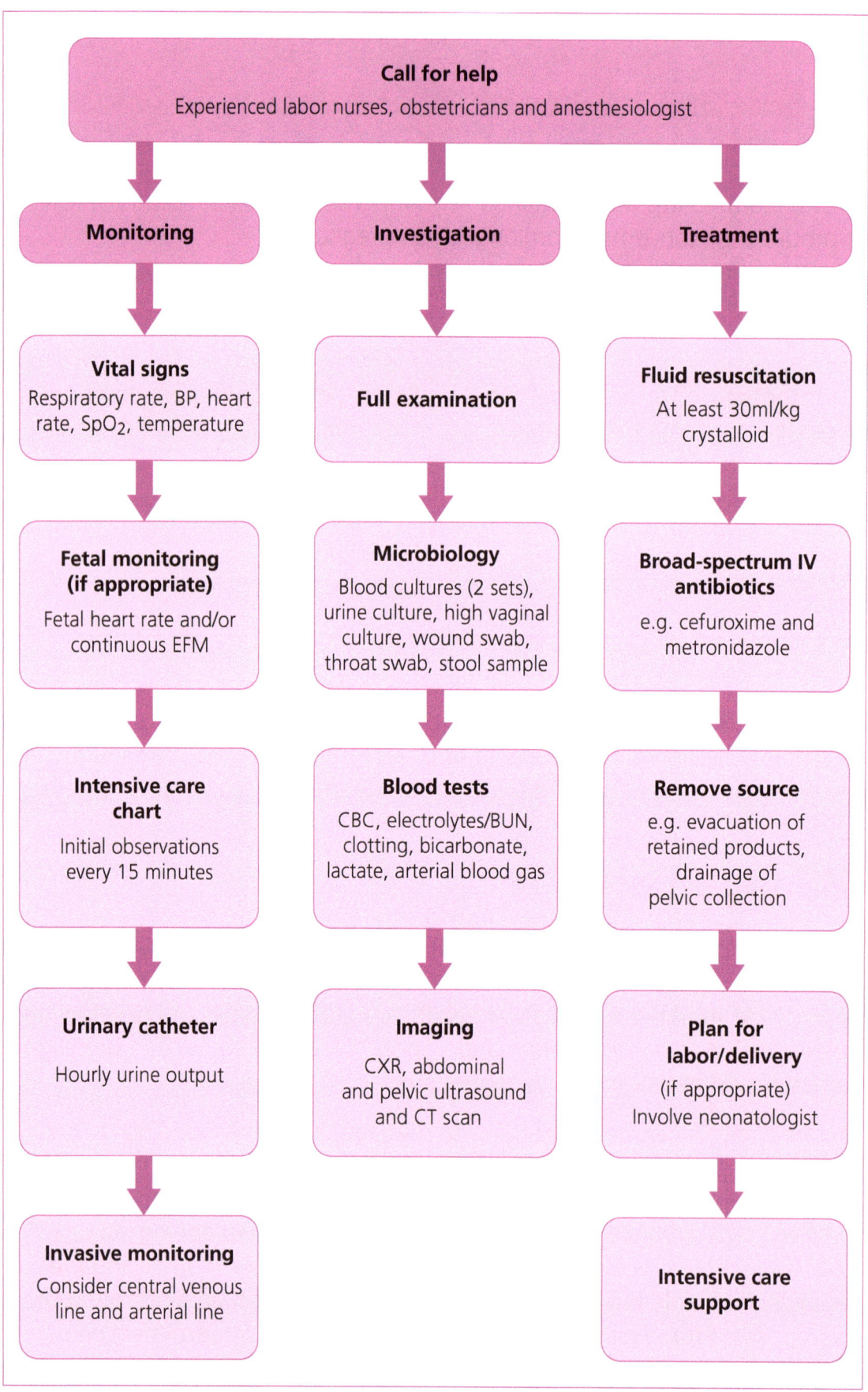

Figure 7.2 Algorithm for the initial management of maternal sepsis

Though the Surviving Sepsis Campaign protocols are detailed, obstetrical management can be reduced to just six steps completed in the first hour after recognition – the so-called Sepsis Six:

1. Give high-flow oxygen and obtain an arterial blood gas if the pulse oximeter oxygen saturation is less than 90%.
2. Take blood cultures.
3. Begin intravenous antibiotics.
4. Start intravenous fluid resuscitation.
5. Take blood samples for hemoglobin and lactate levels.
6. Measure urine output hourly.

After completing these six steps, the patient should be ready to transfer to an appropriate intensity care unit.

Call for help

Early involvement of experienced labor nurses, midwives, obstetricians, anesthesiologists, and critical care physicians is crucial.

Support: airway, breathing, circulation

Monitor and maintain the maternal airway; breathing and circulation are your first priorities. If the woman has collapsed, check that her airway is patent and that she is breathing. Give high-flow oxygen by facemask with a reservoir bag and ensure she stays in the left-lateral position. Secure intravenous access as soon as possible. Obtain an arterial blood gas if the pulse oximeter reading is low.

Prompt early intravenous antibiotic treatment

Immediate high-dose broad-spectrum intravenous antibiotic therapy (e.g., 1.5 g cefuroxime and 500 mg metronidazole), in accordance with local guidelines and practices and known patient allergies, should be initiated as soon as possible.[5] Antibiotic administration should not be delayed until the results of the cultures are available. The blood cultures should be drawn prior to the antibiotics when possible, but do not delay antibiotic treatment in any manner.

If the woman is already extremely ill, deteriorates, or does not improve within 24 hours of treatment, additional or alternative intravenous antibiotics such as gentamicin and clindamycin or piperacillin/tazobactam (Tazocin®; Wyeth) should be used. In such cases, you should consider consultation with the infectious disease service.

Fluid resuscitation

Hypotension and/or an elevated serum lactate level (>4 mmol/l or 36 mg/dl) should be treated with intravenous fluid. Women should be given an initial fluid challenge of 30 ml/kg of intravenous crystalloid.[5] This means a 75 kg patient with sepsis should be given at least 1,500 ml of intravenous crystalloid. If there is no improvement in either her blood pressure and/or the serum lactate level after the fluid bolus, the woman should be transferred to intensive care where vasopressors can be administered to increase and maintain the mean arterial pressure above 65 mmHg.

Full clinical examination

A full clinical examination should be performed with the aim of identifying the cause of the sepsis. This is a head-to-toe examination including a vaginal examination to exclude retained tampons or swabs.

Monitor

Women with sepsis can deteriorate rapidly. Vigilance in observation and assessment is required and vital signs should be recorded on a MOEWS type chart to aid the early detection of a deteriorating patient.

- Respiratory rate, pulse, blood pressure, and oxygen saturations: every 15 minutes until stabilized, then every 30 minutes.
- Temperature measured at least every 4 hours.
- Hourly urine output: Foley catheter with urometer.
- Blood samples every 4 to 12 hours depending on clinical condition: CBC, clotting screen, urea and electrolytes, liver function tests, bicarbonate, and lactate.

Microbiology testing

Cultures should be taken from all potential sources of sepsis. Samples should be sent stat to the microbiology laboratory, where immediate microscopy should be performed on appropriate samples. The results of microbiology testing should be promptly followed up and antibiotic treatment altered accordingly. The samples should include:

- blood cultures (at least two separate sites and from all intravenous cannulas in place longer than 48 hours)
- vaginal swabs
- urine culture
- wound swabs
- throat swab
- stool sample
- sputum sample
- placental swabs (if immediately postpartum).

A common pathogen associated with death from genital tract sepsis is group A beta-hemolytic streptococcus, also known as puerperal sepsis, childbed fever, or Strep A. Other pathogens that commonly cause genital tract sepsis include *Escherichia coli*, group B beta-hemolytic streptococcus, *Staphylococcus aureus*, coagulase-negative staphylococcus, pseudomonas, and mixed anaerobes/bacteroides species. Many women with genital tract sepsis have a mixed infection with two or more organisms.

Blood tests

Complete blood count

The white blood cell count (WBC) in sepsis is commonly greater than 14,000 with a shift left (high band and neutrophil count). However, the WBC may also fall below 4,000, indicating severe sepsis. The platelet count may be low or elevated.

Renal and liver function

Acute tubular necrosis may develop, which can lead to renal failure with raised urea, creatinine, and potassium levels. The pro-inflammatory state of sepsis can also lead to hyperbilirubinemia and jaundice.

Clotting studies

The clinical syndrome of disseminated intravascular coagulation (DIC) is one complication of severe sepsis. The activated partial thromboplastin time (aPTT), prothrombin time, and fibrinogen should be checked. In addition, observe closely for clinical evidence of undue bleeding/bruising. If any of the investigations are abnormal, consider treatment with platelets, fresh frozen plasma (FFP), and/or cryoprecipitate, and consultation with the on-call clinical hematologist as needed.

Serum lactate

Patients with severe sepsis or septic shock typically have a high serum lactate secondary to anaerobic metabolism due to poor tissue perfusion. A lactate level greater than 2 mmol/l is abnormal and a level greater than 4 mmol/l indicates a poor prognosis.[8] Measurement of the lactate level is essential to identify tissue hypoperfusion in patients who are not yet hypotensive but who are at risk of septic shock.

Serum lactate can often be measured by current generations of blood gas analyzers.

Because of the high risk of septic shock, the Surviving Sepsis Campaign recommends any patient with an elevated serum lactate level (>4 mmol/l or 36 mg/dl) be given an initial minimum of 30 ml/kg of crystalloid fluid, regardless of their blood pressure. If there is no improvement in the serum lactate level following the fluid bolus, the patient should be transferred to intensive care for inotropic support.

Arterial blood gas

An arterial blood gas is a fundamental investigation in any patient who is unwell. It is likely to show metabolic acidosis (arterial pH <7.35) due to lactate production. Respiratory compensation may occur in the form of hyperventilation leading to a low $PaCO_2$, but this will never completely correct the low pH. Serum bicarbonate is typically low (normal 24–33 mmol/l) as bicarbonate is consumed in buffering hydrogen ions. As shock progresses, the metabolic acidosis worsens, compensatory mechanisms are exhausted and the blood pH decreases further (<7.20). Early respiratory failure can lead to hypoxia with PaO_2 <60 mmHg.

Remove the source of maternal sepsis

If possible, remove the source of sepsis. Delivery should be expedited if there are signs of chorioamnionitis. Severe maternal infection can also affect the fetus and it is important the pediatric/neonatal staff be fully informed. Any retained products of conception should be removed as soon as the maternal condition is stable. A laparotomy and sometimes hysterectomy may be necessary.

Imaging

Imaging may help to identify the source of the sepsis:

- abdominal ultrasound for retained products of conception or abdominal fluid collection
- chest X-ray
- computed tomography of the chest, abdomen, and pelvis.

Prophylactic treatment

Women with sepsis are at increased risk of venous thromboembolism. Deep venous thrombosis prophylaxis with low-molecular-weight heparin and/or the use of compression stockings are recommended.

Multi-professional approach

Early advice should be sought from other specialists, such as anesthesiologists, intensive care specialists, hematologists, and microbiologists, as well as experienced obstetricians. Critically ill patients should be cared for in an intensive care type unit.

> **There is a need to raise both maternal and professional awareness regarding antenatal, intrapartum, and puerperal sepsis. Local guidelines and protocols should be available to all labor unit and emergency department staff, as well as general practitioners and community midwives, so that maternal sepsis can be promptly recognized and managed.[2]**

References

1. Creanga AA, Berg CJ, Syverson C, Seed K, Bruce FC, Callaghan WM. Pregnancy-related mortality in the United States, 2006–2010. *Obstet Gynecol* 2015; 125(1): 5–12.

2. Centre for Maternal and Child Enquiries. CMACE Emergent Theme Briefing #1: Genital Tract Sepsis. *Saving Mothers' Lives 2006–08: Briefing on genital tract sepsis*. London: CMACE; 2010.

3. Knight M, Kenyon S, Brocklehurst P, Neilson J, Shakespeare J, Kurinczuk JJ (eds) on behalf of MBRRACE UK. *Saving Lives, Improving Mothers' Care: Lessons Learned to Inform Future Maternity Care from the UK and Ireland Confidential Enquiries into Maternal Deaths and Morbidity 2009–12*. Oxford: National Perinatal Epidemiology Unit, University of Oxford; 2014.

4. Betrán AP, Wojdyla D, Posner SF, Gülmezoglu AM. National estimates for maternal mortality: an analysis based on the WHO systematic review of maternal mortality and morbidity. *BMC Public Health* 2005; 5: 131.

5. Sumbul M, Parapia LA. Handwashing and hygiene: lessons from history. *J R Coll Physicians Edinb* 2008; 38: 379.

6. Lewis G (ed.) The Confidential Enquiry into Maternal and Child Health (CEMACH). *Saving Mothers' Lives: Reviewing Maternal Deaths to Make Motherhood Safer 2003–2005. The Seventh Report on Confidential Enquiries into Maternal Deaths in the United Kingdom.* London: CEMACH; 2007.

7. Surviving Sepsis Campaign; 2011 [www.survivingsepsis.org].

8. Weil MH, Afifi AA. Experimental and clinical studies on lactate and pyruvate as indicators of the severity of acute circulatory failure (shock). *Circulation* 1970; 41: 989–1001.

Module 8
Major obstetric hemorrhage

Key learning points

- Understand the main risk factors for and the causes of major obstetric hemorrhage.
- Understand the importance of early recognition of obstetric hemorrhage.
- Be familiar with the immediate management and specific treatment of major antepartum, intrapartum, and postpartum hemorrhage.
- Emphasize the importance of early, adequate fluid resuscitation.
- Communicate effectively with the patient and the multi-professional team.
- Document management accurately, clearly, and legibly.

Common difficulties observed in training drills

- Delayed recognition of the severity of the problem until the woman develops shock.
- Failure to promptly recognize concealed bleeding.
- Not stating the problem clearly to all who attend the emergency.
- Delayed initiation of adequate fluid resuscitation.
- Delayed recognition of the need for operative intervention.

- Uncertainty about how to access blood products rapidly.
- Injudicious use of misoprostol as opposed to other available agents.

Introduction

Massive obstetric hemorrhage is the leading cause of maternal death worldwide, accounting for at least half the deaths in some series.[1] Major obstetric hemorrhage complicates 3.7/1,000 births in the UK,[2] with a maternal mortality of 3.9 per million deliveries.[3] A more recent accounting failed to show further improvement.[4] The corresponding number in the United States is a shocking 90 cases per million deliveries, despite the fact the maternal mortality rate from hemorrhage has declined since 1987.[5] In many series, over half the women who died were judged to have received "major substandard care," implying that if the care had been better, these women would likely have survived.[3] Recurring themes include a lack of early experienced multi-professional involvement, a lack of close postoperative monitoring, failure to act on signs and symptoms, and inadequate use and interpretation of modified obstetric early warning score (MOEWS) charts.

Definition of hemorrhage

Antepartum hemorrhage (APH) is defined as bleeding from the genital tract after the 24th week (sometimes defined as from the 20th week) of pregnancy. It can occur at any time until the onset of labor.

Intrapartum hemorrhage is defined as bleeding from the genital tract at any time during labor until the completion of the 2nd stage of labor.

Primary postpartum hemorrhage (PPH) is traditionally defined as a blood loss of 500 ml or more within the first 24 hours after delivery. However, most healthy women can cope with this amount of blood loss without problems. A major PPH is defined as a blood loss greater than 1,000 ml.[6]

Secondary PPH is defined as a blood loss of 500 ml or more from 24 hours postpartum up until 12 weeks postpartum.[5]

Pathophysiology

The normal adult blood volume approximates 70 ml/kg, which amounts to a total blood volume of about 5 liters. The healthy pregnant woman has a total blood volume of 6 to 7 liters in late pregnancy. This increased blood volume, in conjunction with uterine contraction and raised levels of blood coagulation factors, such as fibrinogen and clotting factors VII, VIII, and X, provide physiological protection against immediate and delayed hemorrhage.

Blood loss can be difficult to estimate and bleeding can be concealed within the uterus, broad ligament, or uterine cavity. Normal blood loss (<500 ml) during a vaginal delivery or during a cesarean delivery does not change the maternal pulse or blood pressure; more significant losses will. Table 8.1 summarizes the clinical features of shock in pregnancy due to the volume of blood loss.

Failure of current practice to take into account maternal stature or weight may account for some underestimates of the magnitude of blood loss. Table 8.2 illustrates the impact of weight.

Clinically apparent coagulopathies may develop as a consequence of severe blood loss. In the clinical syndrome of disseminated intravascular coagulation (DIC), blood is exposed to excessive amounts of clotting factors including thromboplastin. Coagulation factors are consumed rapidly and the fibrinolysis system activated, causing disruption to the control of coagulation balance and fibrinolysis. This may deteriorate until hemostasis is no longer possible.

Table 8.1 Clinical features of shock in pregnancy related to blood loss

Blood loss (ml)	Clinical features	Level of shock
500–1,000	Normal blood pressure, tachycardia, palpitations, dizziness	*Compensated*
1,000–1,500	Hypotension (systolic 90–80 mmHg), tachycardia, tachypnea (21–30 breaths/minute), pale, sweating, weakness, faintness, thirst	*Mild*
1,500–2,000	Hypotension (systolic 80–60 mmHg),a rapid, weak pulse (>110 bpm), tachypnea (>30 breaths/minute), pale, cold clammy skin, poor urinary output (<30 ml/hour), restlessness, anxiety, confusion	*Moderate*
2,000–3,000	Severe hypotension (systolic <50 mmHg), pale, cold, severe clammy skin, peripheral cyanosis, air hunger, anuria, confusion or unconsciousness, collapse	*Severe*

Table 8.2 Estimated blood volumes and proportionate losses according by maternal body weight

Weight	Total blood volume (ml)[a]	15% blood volume loss (ml)	30% blood volume loss (ml)	40% blood volume loss (ml)
50 kg	5,000	750	1,500	2,000
55 kg	5,500	825	1,650	2,200
60 kg	6,000	900	1,800	2,400
65 kg	6,500	975	1,950	2,600
70 kg	7,000	1,050	2,100	2,800

[a]Based on 100 ml/kg blood volume in pregnancy (may overestimate blood volume in obese women).[7,8]

Protocol for major obstetric hemorrhage

All obstetric units should have an obstetric major hemorrhage protocol and the multi-professional team should update and rehearse this protocol regularly in conjunction with hematology and blood bank staff as indicated.[3,4]

Fluid resuscitation

Fluid resuscitation to restore the circulating volume is a priority in any major obstetric hemorrhage.

Fluid resuscitation and administration of blood products are key elements in the management of any major hemorrhage. Maternal blood loss is notoriously difficult to quantify and is often underestimated. Figure 8.1 provides a guide for estimating blood loss. When possible, blood loss should be quantified by weight.

Immediate large intravenous access and fluid replacement

At least two large-bore (14G or 16G) intravenous cannulas should be placed. As the lines are established, blood samples should be withdrawn for CBC, clotting tests, and cross-matching. Crystalloid solutions (e.g., Ringer's solution or 0.9% saline) are the first-line choice for early fluid replacement. Warmed fluids should be infused as rapidly as possible until the systolic blood pressure has been restored.

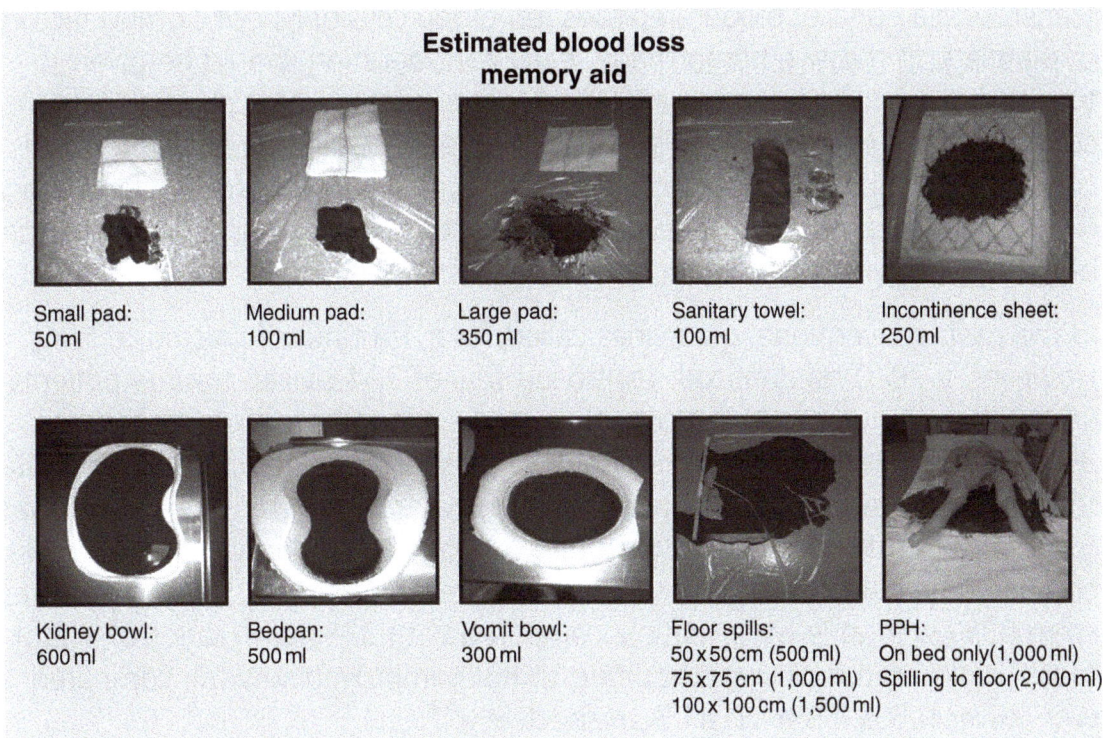

Figure 8.1 An example guide to estimating blood loss.
(S Paterson-Brown model: Bose P, et al. *BJOG* 2006; 113: 919–24)

Volume to be infused

Three liters of clear fluids (crystalloids and colloids) should be administered,[9,10] and consideration given to replacing blood by the most appropriate product (see below).

Give blood and blood products

Intravascular volume and oxygen-carrying capacity need rapid restoration in women with massive hemorrhage. Compatible blood should be transfused as soon as possible (using a blood warmer or rapid infuser). It is preferable to give the mother blood of the same group. However, if fully cross-matched blood is unavailable after three liters of intravenous fluids have been given, or if the bleeding is massive and unrelenting, transfuse O-negative or type-specific blood.

Fluid resuscitation should not be delayed because of a single, reassuring hemoglobin result. Point-of-care tests, such as those for the measurement of hemoglobin (e.g., HemoCue®, HemoCue AB, Ängelholm, Sweden), are vital in cases of massive, rapid hemorrhage because they circumvent the often unavoidable delays in obtaining results of CBCs and clotting screens from the laboratory.

Transfusing a "unit of blood" replaces red blood cells only, not clotting factors or platelets. In massive hemorrhage, early consideration should be given to transfusing fresh frozen plasma (FFP), cryoprecipitate (which provides a more concentrated source of fibrinogen than FFP), and platelet units, all of which contain vital clotting components. It is not necessary to wait for the laboratory results before transfusing these blood products. It is important to contact the blood bank service early.

In the past, conventional guidelines called for a 1:3 ratio of plasma to RBCs. However, a 2010 randomized, controlled trial of 214 civilian trauma patients (in addition to numerous restrospective studies) found significantly higher 30-day survival rates when higher ratios of plasma, platelets, or cryoprecipitate to RBCs were used in patients requiring massive transfusions. The survival was 59% after transfusions with at least one unit of plasma per two of RBCs (1:2), compared with 44% with ratios of 1:3 or more. For platelets, the survival rates were 63% with at least 1:1 ratios, compared with 33% with ratios of 1:2 or more. Higher ratios of cryoprecipitate to RBCs improved survival, compared with lower ratios: 66% vs. 41%, respectively.[11]

Cell salvage

Intraoperative cell salvage (the recovery of blood lost during surgery involving the collection, filtration, washing, and transfusion back into the patient) is commonly used in general surgery and significantly reduces the need for donor blood transfusion. It is increasingly used in obstetrics, especially for women who decline blood or blood products, or when massive blood loss is anticipated (placenta percreta or accreta).[5]

There is a potential for maternal sensitization with cell salvage in rH– women due to contamination with fetal red cells, and the standard dose of anti-D should be given and a Kleihauer test performed one hour after cell salvage has finished to determine whether additional anti-D is required.[4] Care should also be taken to avoid contamination with amniotic fluid.

Antenatal risk assessment for hemorrhage

Anemia

Pre-existing anemia enhances the impact of obstetric hemorrhage, as chronically anemic women are less tolerant of blood loss. Important aspects of antenatal care include antenatal screening of hemoglobin levels and treatment of anemia.

Hemorrhagic disorders

Mothers with inherited hemorrhagic disorders, such as hemophilia and von Willebrand's disease, are at an increased risk of hemorrhage and require specialist care throughout pregnancy, with clear, individualized plans for intrapartum and postpartum management documented in the woman's medical records. Pre-eclampsia complicated by HELLP syndrome (hemolysis, elevated liver enzymes, low platelets) also renders the mother more vulnerable to bleeding.

Placenta previa and accreta

Placenta previa, particularly in women with a prior uterine scar, may be associated with uncontrollable uterine hemorrhage at delivery necessitating cesarean hysterectomy. Experienced obstetricians and anesthesiologists should be drawn upon to plan and perform the cesarean section. Planning should be done prospectively for the use of cell salvage and the potential need of interventional radiology.

Women who decline blood products

Women who may decline blood products should be identified during the antenatal period. A clear plan for the management of potential hemorrhage should be documented in the maternal medical record. This plan should clearly identify specific blood products and treatments that would be acceptable to the woman (including cell salvage), if any. **The principles of the management of hemorrhage are to avoid delay, ensure experienced help is summoned early and to have early access to the use of pharmacological, radiological, and surgical interventions.**[3]

The use of modified obstetric early warning score (MOEWS) charts

It is important to be especially alert to women who are at risk of hemorrhage in order to recognize signs and symptoms of bleeding as early as possible. Several reviews highlight the failure of caregivers to detect the signs and symptoms of intra-abdominal bleeding, particularly after cesarean delivery. We recommend the use of MOEWS charts (Figure 8.2) to address this problem.[3]

The use of the MOEWS chart should alert caregivers to abnormal trends. However, "trigger charts" are useful only if the measurements are accurately plotted and action appropriately taken after alerts. These charts are readily applied to the electronic medical record, which already has graphing capability.

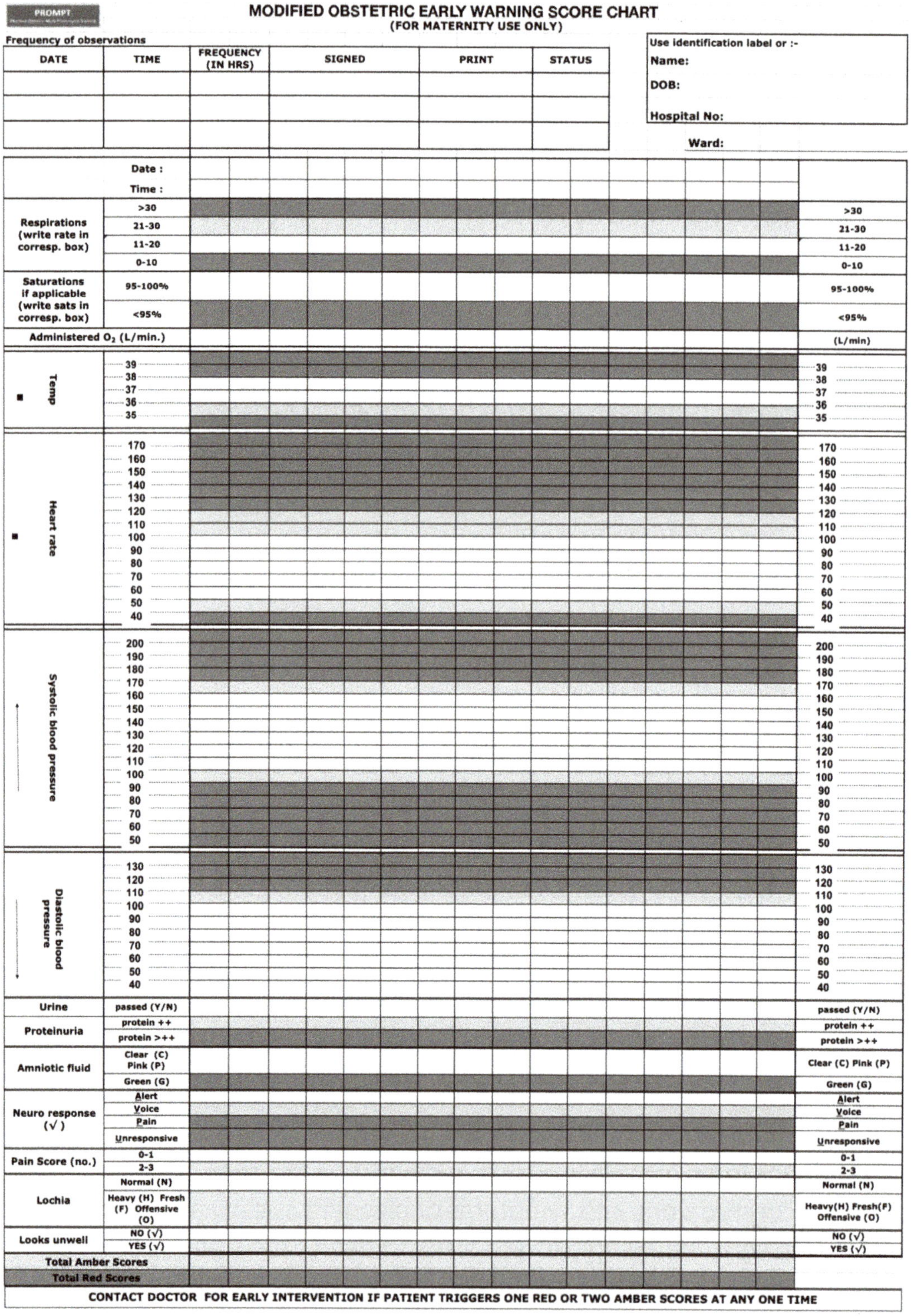

PROMPT

MODIFIED OBSTETRIC EARLY WARNING SCORE CHART
(FOR MATERNITY USE ONLY)

Frequency of observations

DATE	TIME	FREQUENCY (IN HRS)	SIGNED	PRINT	STATUS

Use identification label or :-
Name:
DOB:
Hospital No:
Ward:

	Date :	
	Time :	
Respirations (write rate in corresp. box)	>30	>30
	21-30	21-30
	11-20	11-20
	0-10	0-10
Saturations if applicable (write sats in corresp. box)	95-100%	95-100%
	<95%	<95%
Administered O_2 (L/min.)		(L/min)
Temp	39	39
	38	38
	37	37
	36	36
	35	35
Heart rate	170	170
	160	160
	150	150
	140	140
	130	130
	120	120
	110	110
	100	100
	90	90
	80	80
	70	70
	60	60
	50	50
	40	40
Systolic blood pressure	200	200
	190	190
	180	180
	170	170
	160	160
	150	150
	140	140
	130	130
	120	120
	110	110
	100	100
	90	90
	80	80
	70	70
	60	60
	50	50
Diastolic blood pressure	130	130
	120	120
	110	110
	100	100
	90	90
	80	80
	70	70
	60	60
	50	50
	40	40
Urine	passed (Y/N)	passed (Y/N)
Proteinuria	protein ++	protein ++
	protein >++	protein >++
Amniotic fluid	Clear (C) Pink (P)	Clear (C) Pink (P)
	Green (G)	Green (G)
Neuro response (√)	Alert	Alert
	Voice	Voice
	Pain	Pain
	Unresponsive	Unresponsive
Pain Score (no.)	0-1	0-1
	2-3	2-3
Lochia	Normal (N)	Normal (N)
	Heavy (H) Fresh (F) Offensive (O)	Heavy(H) Fresh(F) Offensive (O)
Looks unwell	NO (√)	NO (√)
	YES (√)	YES (√)
Total Amber Scores		
Total Red Scores		

CONTACT DOCTOR FOR EARLY INTERVENTION IF PATIENT TRIGGERS ONE RED OR TWO AMBER SCORES AT ANY ONE TIME

Reproduced with kind permission of the Aberdeen Maternity Hospital. Ref: CEMACH: 2003-05 and also North Bristol NHS Trust

Figure 8.2 An example of a MOEWS chart and guidance for use

Antepartum hemorrhage

Antepartum hemorrhage complicates 2 to 5% of all pregnancies.[12] It is often unpredictable, and the woman's condition may deteriorate rapidly before, during, or after the onset of hemorrhage.

Causes of APH

The most common causes of minor APH are marginal placental bleeds, bleeding from a cervical ectropion, or a blood-stained "show," which is a product of cervical dilation. The most common causes of *major* APH are placental abruption and placenta previa. Uterine rupture (secondary to the forces of labor, or abdominal trauma including motor vehicle accidents) can also produce massive hemorrhage.

Ruptured vasa previa may cause catastrophic APH for the fetus. Although ruptured vasa previa is not associated with major maternal blood loss, it is an obstetric emergency owing to the rapid development of acute fetal anemia.

Clinical presentation of major APH

A woman with an APH usually presents with obvious vaginal bleeding; however, bleeding may be concealed. The possibility of hemorrhage must be considered in any pregnant women with signs or symptoms of shock or a history of collapse.

Table 8.3 lists the presenting features and causes of APH.

Initial management of major APH

Major APH is an obstetric emergency. Blood loss can be torrential with rapid deterioration in both the maternal and fetal condition. Remember that blood loss is often underestimated and may be concealed, especially in the case of uterine rupture or placental abruption.

The management of a major APH requires the prompt initiation of multiple, simultaneous actions. Rapid assessment of fetal and maternal wellbeing is required. The first step is to stabilize the mother regardless of cause, followed by cause-specific treatment. The exact sequence will be dictated by the needs of the individual patient, her fetus, and the resources available.

An outline of the initial management for a major APH is shown in Figure 8.3. This is discussed in more detail in the following section.

Table 8.3 Presenting features and causes of APH

Cause	Possible presenting features	Condition of uterus	Condition of fetus	Risk factors/ contributory factors
Placenta previa	Painless vaginal bleeding High presenting part or transverse lie Shock	Non-tender and soft or irritable uterus	Reflects the amount of maternal blood loss	Previous uterine surgery, e.g., cesarean section Low-lying placenta on antenatal ultrasound
Placental abruption	Bleeding (may be concealed) Constant pain Fetal compromise Abnormal FHR Maternal shock	Tender, woody, hard uterus or irritable uterus	Dependent on maternal blood loss and duration since abruption occurred	Previous abruption (up to 1:4 recurrence risk if two prior abruptions)[13] Pre-eclampsia, hypertension IUGR Cocaine use Smoking Abdominal trauma Advanced maternal age Grand multiparty
Uterine rupture	Sudden onset of constant sharp pain Peritoneal signs Abnormal FHR Very high or unreachable presenting part Bleeding (may be concealed) Shock Hematuria	Contractions may cease	Likely to have an abnormal FHR Fetal parts palpated outside the uterus	Previous uterine surgery (cesarean section/ myomectomy/corneal ectopic pregnancy) $\geq$4 parity Trauma Oxytocin infusion
Vasa previa	Variable fresh vaginal bleeding after membrane rupture Acute fetal compromise No maternal shock	Normal	Acute fetal compromise – sinusoidal/ bradycardia Fetal mortality 33–100%	Low-lying placenta Succenturiate lobe

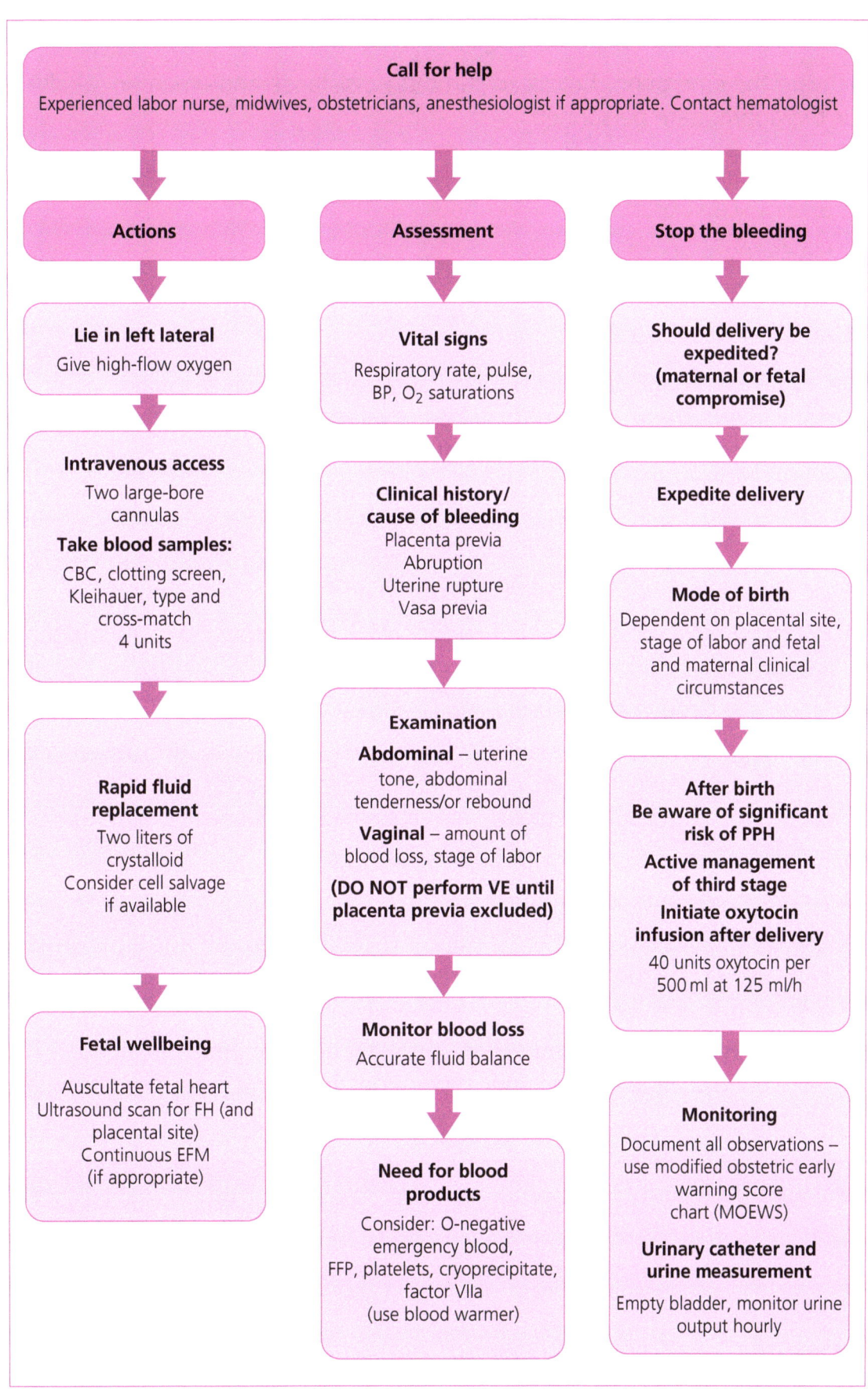

Figure 8.3 Algorithm for the initial management of major APH

Call for help

Activate the emergency buzzer to summon assistance and emergency call for the appropriate personnel:

- senior labor nurse or midwife
- experienced obstetrician
- experienced anesthesiologist
- experienced neonatologist
- additional support staff.

Alert the blood bank, operating room, and transport that the major obstetric hemorrhage protocol may be activated. The senior obstetrician and anesthesiologist should also be informed.

Actions

- Lie the woman in the left-lateral position and give high-flow oxygen.
- Record pulse, blood pressure, capillary refill, respiratory rate, and oxygen saturations.
- Place two large intravenous cannulas.
- Stat blood samples: CBC, Kleihauer (if woman is rhesus-negative), coagulation studies including fibrinogen, cross-match 4 units of blood (consider requesting group-specific blood until cross-matched blood is available).
- Rapid fluid resuscitation with 2 liters of crystalloid.
- Assess need for blood products.
- Use O-negative blood if there is a life-threatening hemorrhage and consider early use of coagulation products, especially if operative delivery is indicated.
- Assess fetal wellbeing – auscultate the fetal heart or perform an ultrasound scan and commence continuous electronic fetal monitoring if appropriate.

> **Ultrasonography is unreliable for the detection of an abruption; time should not be wasted attempting to identify a retroplacental clot using ultrasound scanning.**

Assessment – rapid evaluation of maternal and fetal condition

Quickly assess the overall condition of the mother and fetus.

- Ascertain relevant obstetric and clinical history, including:
  - ☐ gestational age
  - ☐ prior uterine surgery/cesarean section
  - ☐ placental location (refer to any antenatal scans)
  - ☐ abdominal pain.
- Examination:
  - ☐ estimate blood loss (see Figure 8.1)
  - ☐ assess uterine tone and tenderness
  - ☐ palpate the abdomen for peritoneal signs and *ex utero* fetal parts
  - ☐ assess placental site using ultrasound scan
  - ☐ once placenta previa is excluded, perform a speculum examination to assess degree of bleeding and possible local causes (trauma, polyps, ectropion); consider a vaginal examination to ascertain stage of labor.

> **Do not perform a vaginal examination in the presence of vaginal bleeding without first excluding placenta previa.**

Stop the bleeding – should delivery be initiated?

In women with massive APH, delivery is the most effective method of controlling the bleeding, irrespective of the cause, and can be a life-saving intervention for the mother.[8] If there is a placenta previa, removal of the abnormally implanted placenta should control the bleeding, but the team must remain alert to the high risk of major PPH. The most experienced obstetrician available should perform the operative delivery.

If APH is caused by uterine rupture, the site should be identified and repaired if appropriate. Regardless of the suspected fetal compromise, the maternal condition should always take precedence. If delivery is indicated (irrespective of gestation), the mother should be appropriately resuscitated, and the birth expedited. It should not be delayed for fetal reasons, such as waiting for steroid effect in cases of prematurity.

The neonatal team should be notified early in cases of major APH, to ensure adequate time to prepare neonatal resuscitation equipment. Antepartum hemorrhage can cause neonatal anemia, particularly when there is vasa previa or less commonly abruption.

It is likely that in cases of major APH delivery will be by emergency cesarean section unless the woman is in labor and fully dilated. A cesarean delivery for major APH (whether caused by an abruption, previa, or uterine rupture) is likely to be technically difficult and should be performed by the most experienced obstetrician available.

The choice of anesthetic for an operative procedure will depend on the clinical circumstances and maternal condition and should be decided by an experienced anethesiologist.

Finally, an APH is a major risk factor for PPH, and all members of the team should be prepared.

Postpartum hemorrhage

Major PPH (>1,000 ml) complicates 1 to 2% of deliveries.[14] The clinical features of shock are as previously described in Table 8.1. Major PPH is an obstetric emergency.

Risk factors for major PPH

Prelabor and intrapartum risk factors for PPH are listed in Box 8.1.

Prevention of PPH

There is a strong evidence base to support routine active management of the 3rd stage of labor to limit PPH.[15] A combination of oxytocin and methylergonovine reduces the risk of PPH by 60%. However, methylergonovine is associated with postpartum hypertension, nausea, and vomiting. Oxytocin (10 units IM or 5 units IV) alone is considered by some authorities to be the agent of choice for women without risk factors for PPH.[4] It is not associated with postpartum hypertension and therefore should be used alone instead of with methylergonovine in the presence of maternal hypertension or if the maternal blood pressure is not known prior to delivery.[16]

> **Methylergonovine should not be administered in the presence of known hypertension or if the maternal blood pressure has not been taken during labor.**

Uterine atony should be anticipated in clinical situations such as prolonged labor or 2nd-stage cesarean section. In high-risk cases, consider administering an infusion of oxytocin 40 units in 500 ml 0.9% saline intravenously (125 ml/hour) for up to 4 hours after birth in addition to methylergonovine (200 mcg) (if appropriate).

The placental site should be determined by ultrasound in all women with a prior cesarean section, and if the placenta is low, magnetic resonance imaging (MRI)

Box 8.1 Risk factors for PPH

Prelabor

Prior retained placenta or PPH (recurrence rate of about 8–10%)

Placenta previa, accreta or percreta

Prior cesarean delivery (associated with placenta previa, percreta, and accreta)

Antepartum hemorrhage – especially from placental abruption

Overdistension of uterus (e.g., multiple pregnancy, polyhydramnios, macrosomia)

Pre-eclampsia

Body mass index >35

Increased maternal age (older women are less tolerant to the effects of a massive bleed)

Existing uterine abnormalities (e.g., fibroids)

Maternal anemia (<9 g/dl at start of labor) (less able to tolerate hemorrhage)

Grand multiparity

Intrapartum

Induction of labor

Prolonged 1st, 2nd, or 3rd stage of labor

Oxytocin use in labor

Retained placenta

Precipitate labor

Operative vaginal birth

Cesarean delivery, particularly in the 2nd stage of labor

Placental abruption

Fever in labor

used together with ultrasound to attempt to determine whether there is an accreta or percreta. A detailed plan should be placed in the antenatal record if either is confirmed, as the involvement of an experienced multi-disciplinary team at delivery may prevent or reduce the risk of intrapartum and postpartum hemorrhage.[3,4]

Causes of PPH

Major PPH usually occurs within the first hour after delivery, hence the reason a 4-hour oxytocin infusion is so effective. The most common cause is uterine atony (70–90%), with or without retained placental tissue.

Genital tract trauma is the second most common cause of PPH, followed by coagulation defects, which are rare but an occasional cause of significant hemorrhage. Table 8.4 lists some of the presenting features, which may be accompanied by signs and symptoms of shock. It is important to remember that the bleeding may be totally or partially concealed. Concealed hemorrhage should be suspected when the observations and estimated blood loss do not tally. Rupture of the uterus usually occurs before or at birth, but the diagnosis may not be made until after birth.

Placenta percreta or accreta is typically diagnosed when massive hemorrhage follows an unsuccessful attempt to remove the placenta. One case-control study of peripartum hysterectomy reported that 39% of the women requiring peripartum hysterectomy for hemorrhage had either percreta or accreta.[17]

Initial management of major PPH

The management of a major PPH requires the prompt initiation of multiple simultaneous actions in a sequence similar to APH. The exact sequence will be dictated by the needs of the individual patient and the resources available.

Table 8.4 Presenting features and causes of PPH

Presenting feature	Condition of uterus	Possible cause
Vaginal bleeding, placenta delivered complete	"Boggy" and high	Uterine atony
Vaginal bleeding, placenta delivered incomplete	"Boggy" and high	Retained placental tissue
Vaginal bleeding, placenta delivered complete	Well contracted	Vaginal/cervical/ perineal trauma
Symptoms of shock, often without vaginal bleeding	At the vulva and not palpable abdominally	Inverted uterus
Continual bleeding, blood not clotting, oozing from wound sites	"Boggy" or contracted	Coagulopathy

An outline of the initial management for a major PPH is shown in Figure 8.4. This is discussed in more detail in the following section.

Call for help

Activate the emergency buzzer to call for assistance:

- senior-most labor nurse or midwife
- experienced obstetrician
- additional support staff
- anesthesiologist
- transport volunteer ready to take urgent samples.

Alert the blood bank and operating room staff to be on standby in the event that the major obstetric hemorrhage protocol is activated.

Postpartum hemorrhage emergency box

For those units that do not use a computerized unit for drug distribution and storage, a PPH emergency box (Figure 8.5) containing emergency equipment, treatment algorithms, and medication required for the immediate management of PPH may be helpful.

Immediate actions – irrespective of cause

- Lie the woman flat and give high-flow oxygen by facemask.
- **Vigorous** uterine massage to expel any clots from the uterus.
- Place two large bore intravenous cannulas and send stat blood samples: CBC, coagulation studies including fibrinogen, and cross-match for 4 units of blood (if appropriate, request group-specific blood until cross-matched blood available).
- Rapid infusion of at least 2 liters of crystalloid (e.g. Ringer's solution or normal saline).
- Autotransfuse the patient by elevating her legs and/or head-down tilt.
- Use O-negative blood in cases of life-threatening hemorrhage.

Assessment – rapid evaluation

Quickly assess the overall condition of the mother. This includes:

- pulse, blood pressure, respiratory rate, and oxygen saturations

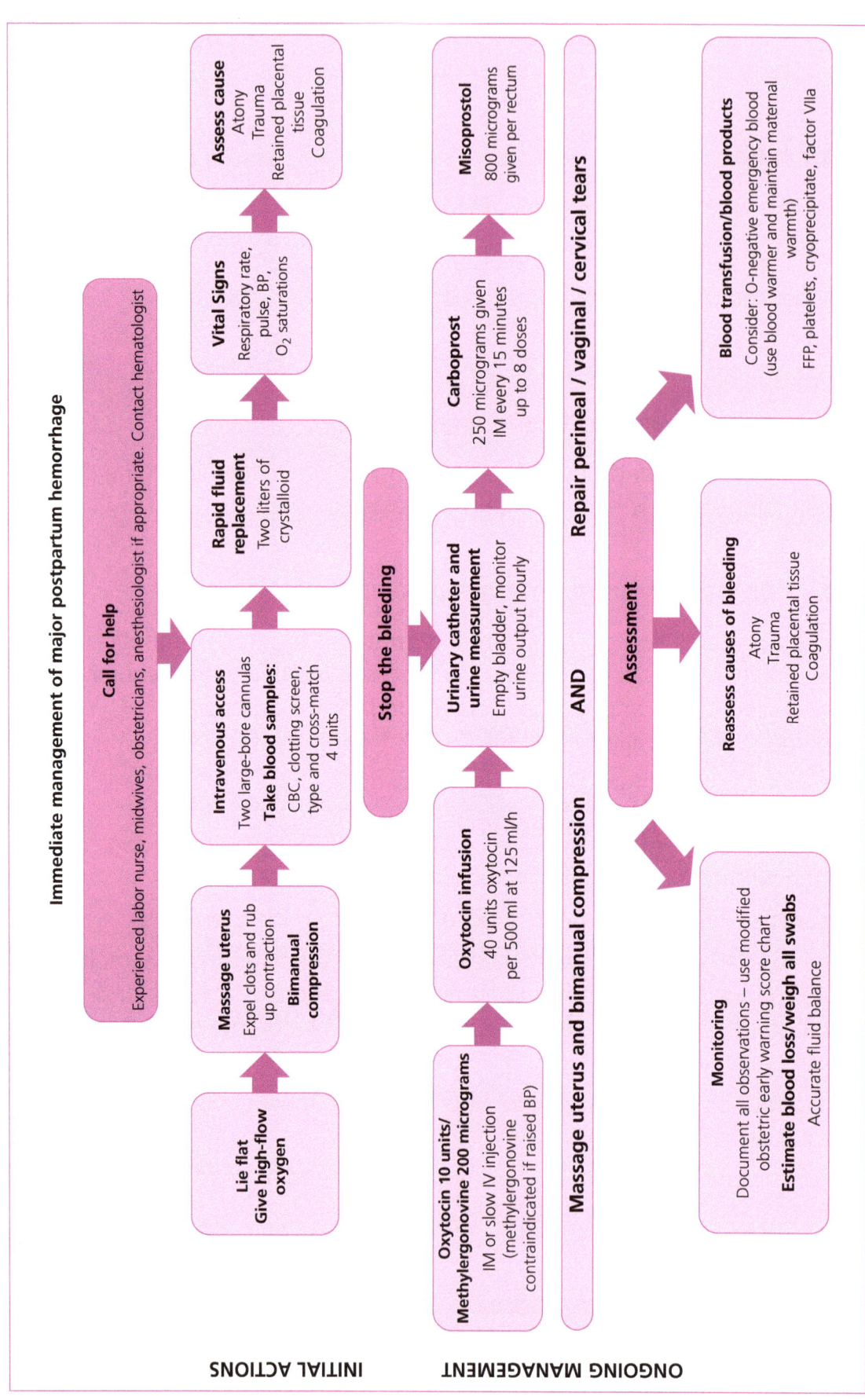

Immediate management of major postpartum hemorrhage

Call for help

Experienced labor nurse, midwives, obstetricians, anesthesiologist if appropriate. Contact hematologist

INITIAL ACTIONS

Lie flat
Give high-flow oxygen

Massage uterus
Expel clots and rub up contraction
Bimanual compression

Intravenous access
Two large-bore cannulas
Take blood samples:
CBC, clotting screen, type and cross-match 4 units

Rapid fluid replacement
Two liters of crystalloid

Vital Signs
Respiratory rate, pulse, BP, O_2 saturations

Assess cause
Atony
Trauma
Retained placental tissue
Coagulation

ONGOING MANAGEMENT

Stop the bleeding

Oxytocin 10 units/
Methylergonovine 200 micrograms
IM or slow IV injection
(methylergonovine contraindicated if raised BP)

Oxytocin infusion
40 units oxytocin per 500 ml at 125 ml/h

Urinary catheter and urine measurement
Empty bladder, monitor urine output hourly

Carboprost
250 micrograms given IM every 15 minutes up to 8 doses

Misoprostol
800 micrograms given per rectum

Massage uterus and bimanual compression

AND

Repair perineal / vaginal / cervical tears

Assessment

Monitoring
Document all observations – use modified obstetric early warning score chart
Estimate blood loss/weigh all swabs
Accurate fluid balance

Reassess causes of bleeding
Atony
Trauma
Retained placental tissue
Coagulation

Blood transfusion/blood products
Consider: O-negative emergency blood (use blood warmer and maintain maternal warmth)
FFP, platelets, cryoprecipitate, factor VIIa

Figure 8.4 Algorithm for the initial management of a major PPH

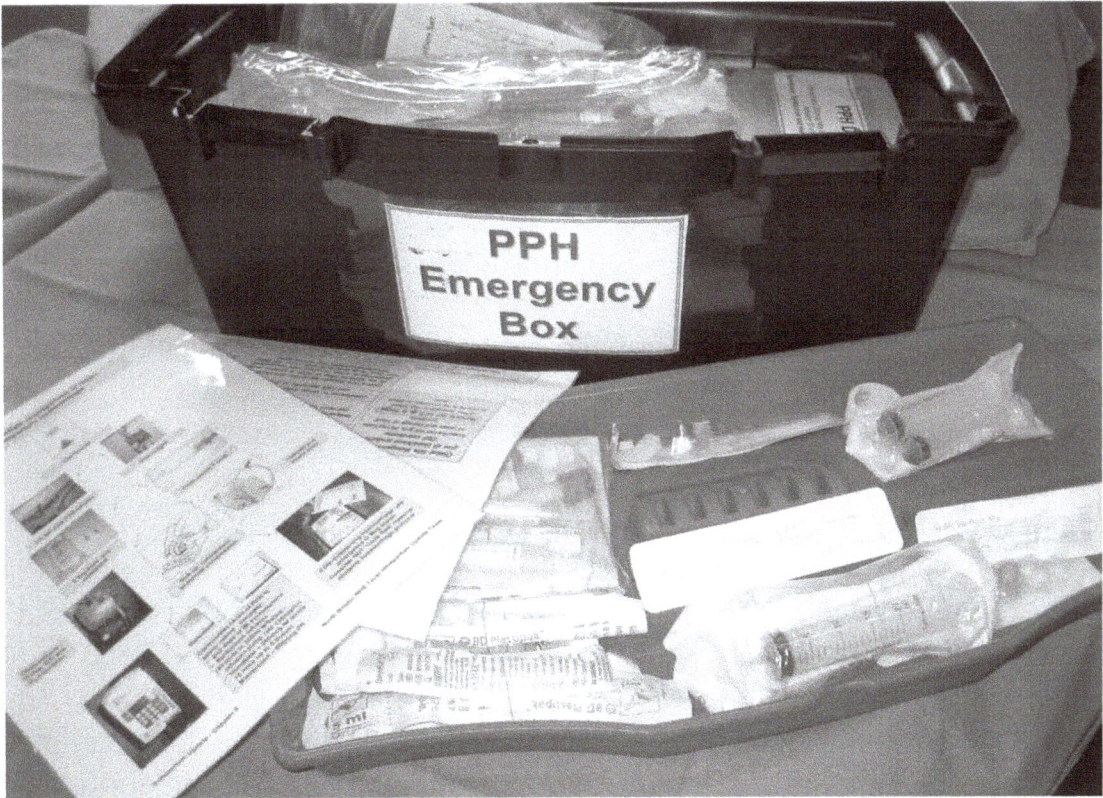

Figure 8.5 The postpartum hemorrhage emergency box

- peripheral perfusion
- check uterine tone
- estimate blood loss: weigh swabs, incontinence pads, etc.

Observe for signs of shock:

- maternal tachycardia of greater than 100 beats/minute
- respiratory rate of over 30 breaths/minute
- peripheral vasoconstriction.

All indicate significant blood loss with initial physiological compensation (see Table 8.1). If the systolic blood pressure falls below 100 mmHg, the blood loss is likely to be at least 25% of the maternal blood volume.

Try to identify the cause:

- Check whether the uterus is well contracted.
- Check that the placenta has been expelled and is complete.
- Examine the cervix, vagina, and perineum for tears – again!
- Observe for signs of clotting disorders, such as oozing from wound and puncture sites.

Stop the bleeding

Remember there may be more than one cause for the bleeding.

Massage the uterus

The most common cause of PPH is uterine atony. Check that the uterus is well contracted. If the uterus is flaccid, massage vigorously until it is firm. This is not a time to be dainty. Expel any trapped blood clots, as these inhibit effective contractions. Use bimanual compression if bleeding continues.

First-line drug therapy

If the 3rd stage of labor was not actively managed, give either 10 units oxytocin intramuscularly or 5 units intravenously. If the blood pressure is not elevated, you can improve efficacy by adding methylergonovine 0.2 mg intramuscular, depending on clinical circumstances and availability. If an oxytocic has already been given for active management of the 3rd stage but bleeding is continuing, give a second dose of oxytocin as outlined above.

> **Use caution with repeated bolus doses of intravenous oxytocin when there is maternal hypotension, as oxytocin can cause a further fall in blood pressure.[18]**

If the uterus contracts with the measures outlined above, begin an oxytocin infusion (40 units diluted in 500 ml normal saline) over 4 hours to maintain uterine tone. However, if the uterine tone is poor, other treatments (e.g., expulsion of blood clots or removal of retained placental tissue) will be necessary before the oxytocin infusion will be effective.

Catheterize the bladder

Some believe a full bladder can inhibit effective contraction of the uterus. Inserting a Foley catheter to empty the bladder eliminates that possibility and facilitates the monitoring of maternal renal function.

Repair any tears

Vaginal tears are the second most frequent cause of PPH. Apply pressure to minimize blood loss. Stabilize the mother and repair any tears as soon as possible, ensuring adequate analgesia and good lighting. Consider early transfer to the operating room, as a full examination under anesthesia is often required for adequate visualization.

Continuing bleeding

Most cases of hemorrhage are successfully controlled by the simple measures outlined above: a second dose of oxytocin, bladder catheterization, and repair of vaginal tears. However, in some cases the bleeding will continue and further management is required. Such management is most effectively performed in the operating room.

Bimanual compression of the uterus

Bimanual massage of the uterus should be vigorously performed if the bleeding continues (Figure 8.6) while the woman is transferred to the operating room. It is an excellent holding measure and should be continued until the hemorrhage is brought under control.

Gently insert one hand into the vagina and form a fist. Direct your fist into the anterior fornix and apply pressure against the anterior wall of the uterus. With the other hand, press externally on the uterine fundus and compress the uterus between your hands. Maintain the compression until bleeding is controlled and the uterus contracts. Whether in the community setting or on a postpartum ward, bimanual compression provides an effective mechanical holding measure until arrival back in the labor suite.

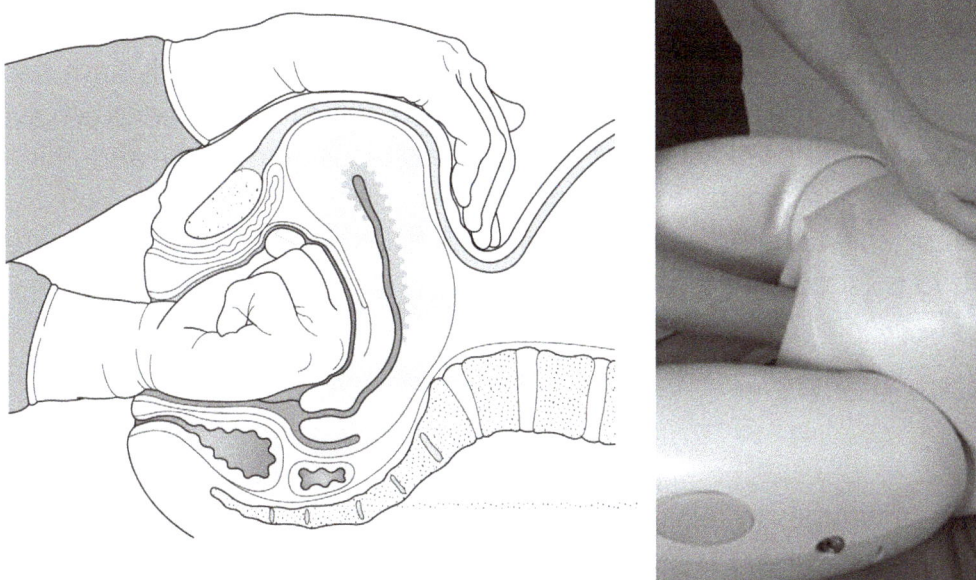

Figure 8.6 Bimanual compression of the uterus

Examination under anesthetic

There should be a low threshold for examination under anesthesia. Adequate exposure is essential.

Manual removal of retained products

Persistent uterine atony is often caused by retained blood clots or placental tissue. Exploration and emptying of the uterus should be performed as soon as the mother has been resuscitated. This is best performed in the operating room. When the uterus has been manually explored and emptied, additional oxytocics should be administered to contract the uterus.

Repair of cervical, vaginal, and perineal tears

Adequate analgesia, good lighting, and a surgical assistant make the identification and repair of genital tract tears easier. A systematic approach should be used to ensure that no tears (especially high vaginal and cervical tears) are missed during suturing.

Treatment of unrelenting hemorrhage

Emptying the uterus, giving simple uterotonics, and suturing any tears will control almost all cases of hemorrhage. Should bleeding continue despite these actions, further management will be required as continuation poses a significant threat to the life of the mother.

In cases of unrelenting hemorrhage, both bimanual compression and aortic compression can be used to stem the bleeding until other methods have had time to take effect. The aorta must be compressed against the spine to achieve compression. Use a closed fist to apply downward pressure over the abdominal aorta just above and slightly to the left of the umbilicus (Figure 8.7). You should not be able to palpate the femoral pulse if the compression is adequate. This method is especially useful if the PPH occurs during a cesarean section.

Drug treatments

Carboprost

If the uterus continues to relax despite initial measures, give carboprost (Hemabate®, Pharmacia) 250 mcg by deep intramuscular injection. This can be repeated at 15-minute intervals for a maximum of eight doses. Adverse effects are uncommon but include vomiting, diarrhea, headache, hypertension, and

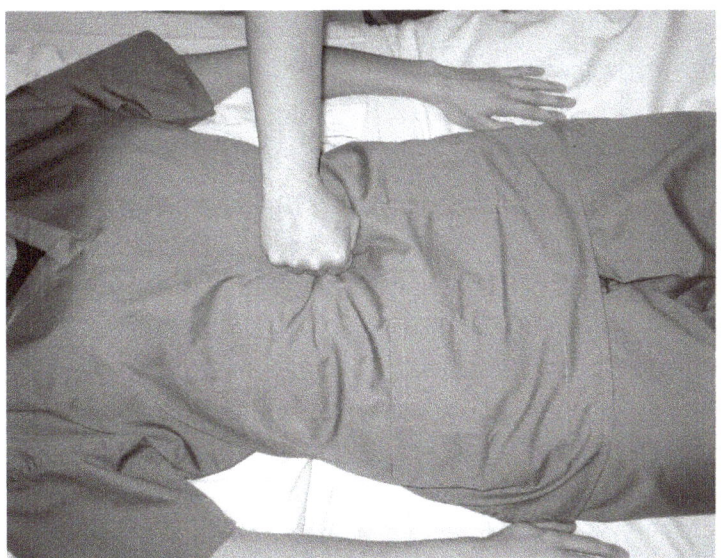

Figure 8.7 Aortic compression

bronchospasm. Carboprost is contraindicated in women with cardiac or pulmonary disease, including asthma.

> **Do not give carboprost intravenously. Prostaglandins can be fatal if given intravenously.**

Misoprostol

The use of rectal misoprostol (800–1,000 mcg) has been described. Misoprostol is a synthetic analogue of prostaglandin E1 and has the advantage of being thermostable and inexpensive. A systematic review of the prophylactic use of oral misoprostol for the management of the 3rd stage of labor found that misoprostol 600 mcg was less effective than conventional oxytocin and methylergonovine when used individually.[19,20] It may be of benefit in addition to oxytocin in place of methylergonovine. Misoprostol may also be used if 1st- and 2nd-line uterotonics (e.g., oxytocin, ergometrine, and carboprost) are unavailable or contraindicated.[4]

Tranexamic acid

Tranexamic acid is an antifibrinolytic used widely to prevent and treat hemorrhage in non-obstetric patients. A systematic review published in 2010 suggests that 0.5 g or 1 g tranexamic acid intravenously decreases postpartum blood loss after vaginal birth and after cesarean section.[21] Further investigations are needed to confirm the efficacy and safety of this regimen. The WOMAN (World Maternal Antifibrinolytic) trial is currently under way seeking to provide reliable evidence as to whether tranexamic acid reduces mortality, hysterectomy, and other morbidities in women with clinically diagnosed PPH.[22]

Recombinant factor VIIa

Recombinant factor VIIa (rFVIIa) was originally developed for patients with hemophilia. Recombinant factor VIIa results in hemostasis by enhancing thrombin generation leading to a stable fibrin clot that is resistant to premature fibrinolysis. Subsequently, it has been used to treat massive intraoperative hemorrhage. Recombinant factor VIIa has also been used successfully in obstetrics to control hemorrhage,[23] though there is a high rate of thromboembolic events in patients who receive it. Therefore rFVIIa should be used with caution and only after consultation with a hematologist. Further, rFVIIa is not effective when the platelets and fibrinogen are very low (below 20×10^9/l and 1 g/l, respectively). The recommended dose is between 40 and 90 mcg/kg.[4,18]

Mechanical and surgical measures

Uterine packing/tamponade

Uterine packing involves the complete and uniform packing of the uterine cavity with mesh gauze. The pack can be inserted inside a sterile plastic drape for easier removal. The evidence from many case reports over several decades suggests that uterine packing is useful for the control of hemorrhage, with few reports of infection or adverse events.[24]

Uterine balloon tamponade (e.g., Bakri [© Cook Medical] or Rusch balloon) can be used in preference to gauze packing. The balloon catheter is inserted into the uterine cavity and inflated with approximately 500 ml of warm saline. An oxytocin infusion is initiated to maintain uterine contraction. This method is described as the "tamponade test."[25] If the tamponade test fails to stop the bleeding (after a vaginal delivery), a laparotomy is indicated. The balloon can be left in place for up to 24 hours. Ideally, it should be removed during the day when the most experienced staff are likely to be available in case bleeding recurs.[4]

Laparotomy

A laparotomy may be needed so that surgical methods can be used in an attempt to stop the bleeding. There are numerous options; no particular surgical procedure can be recommended over another for the treatment of PPH.[26]

B-Lynch suture and other compression measures

The B-Lynch suture technique is simple and effective with successful outcomes in a number of case reports.[4,27] However, it is not a panacea; in one survey, 16% of peripartum hysterectomies performed in the UK were preceded by an unsuccessful B-Lynch or other brace suture.[12]

A simple diagram of the B-Lynch technique is shown in Figure 8.8. The original description of the technique requires the uterine cavity to be opened and explored and a bimanual compression test employed prior to insertion of the suture. *If bimanual compression is ineffective in reducing the bleeding, the B-Lynch suture is unlikely to be successful.*

Several modifications of the B-Lynch suture are described. They all follow the same principle of compressing the uterus to stop the bleeding. Some techniques do not require opening of the uterine cavity, while others describe parallel or vertical sutures that compress the anterior uterine wall against the posterior wall.[4] Most of the published series have favorable outcomes, with subsequent pregnancies reported after the procedure. However, serious complications including uterine necrosis[28] and uterine rupture in a subsequent pregnancy[29] are also reported.

Interventional radiology

Interventional radiology should be considered in high-risk cases (e.g., cases of placenta previa with accreta) where intra-arterial balloons can be placed immediately prior to a planned cesarean section.[4] The technique is often difficult to perform in an emergency situation owing to the specialized equipment and

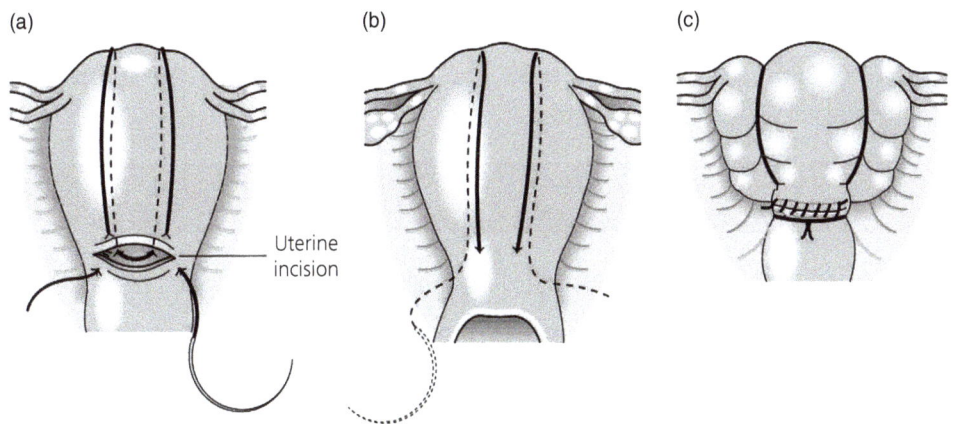

Figure 8.8 The B-Lynch suture: (a) and (b) illustrate the anterior and posterior views of the uterus as the brace suture is placed; (c) shows the anatomical appearance after complete application. (Original illustration by Mr. Philip Wilson FMAA AIMI, based on the author's video record of the operation; reproduced with permission from *Br J Obstet Gynaecol* 1997; 104: 374)

personnel required. As a result, other techniques (e.g., uterine balloon tamponade or compression sutures) may be more appropriate. Interventional radiology can be particularly useful if there is prolonged or continuous bleeding, once initial treatment has been given and the mother is stable for transfer.

Uterine vessel and internal iliac artery ligation

The uterine ovarian and internal iliac vessels can all be ligated in an attempt to stem uterine bleeding. These are potentially difficult procedures and those inexperienced in the technique should seek the assistance of a vascular surgeon if possible.

It is impossible to assess which of the various "surgical" hemostatic techniques is most effective. Nevertheless, the available observational data suggest that balloon tamponade and hemostatic suturing (e.g., B-Lynch) may be more effective than internal iliac artery ligation and are also easier to perform.[4]

Hysterectomy

Hysterectomy may be necessary if bleeding persists. The total incidence of peripartum hysterectomy in the UK in 2005 to 2006 was 41/100,000 births.[12] It was dramatically higher in the United States: about 25 per 100,000 deliveries for atony and 401 per 100,000 including placental abnormalities.[30] It is good practice to involve a second experienced physician in the decision for hysterectomy;[4] however, this should not result in unnecessary delay. Furthermore, this course of action should not be delayed by attempts with other unfamiliar techniques.

Unrelenting hemorrhage is probably one of the most challenging situations in obstetrics. While the decision to perform a hysterectomy is never taken lightly, it is important not to delay this course of action until the mother is moribund or her clotting ability has deteriorated.

Continuing management key points

- Carboprost by deep intramuscular injection
- Use manual holding measures while arranging further treatment
- Invasive monitoring
- Early recourse to surgical intervention
- Watch out for consumptive coagulopathy
- Hysterectomy is life saving and should not be delayed
- Aftercare in high-dependency or intensive care unit

Documentation and obstetric critical care

It is important the woman's clinical response to fluid replacement and the measures performed to control hemorrhage are regularly observed, documented, and evaluated. There should be continuous monitoring of respirations, pulse rate, blood pressure, and oxygenation. The volume and type of fluid administered should be documented so her fluid balance can be easily calculated. Maternal temperature should be monitored as hypothermia can easily develop after the administration of non-warmed blood products.

Clinical observations and fluid balance should be plotted on a critical care chart, which includes modified obstetric early warning scores for early recognition of any deterioration in condition.[3]

Obstetric critical care

Women who have experienced major obstetric hemorrhage (antepartum or postpartum) that causes maternal compromise require high-dependency care. A central line should be considered early to help guide fluid replacement.[3] This is particularly useful when major hemorrhage occurs in a woman with pre-eclampsia, where there is a fine balance between fluid replacement and fluid overload.

Some women may need to be transferred to an intensive care unit, either because of a need for specialist monitoring/therapy or if labor staff are unable to deliver the required care. It is important for the multi-professional team to involve intensivists at an early stage so as to prevent delay in transfer. The use of a maternal SBAR form may aid the communication process for transfer between the labor floor and ICU (see Module 1, Figure 1.1).

References

1. Khan KS, Wojdyla D, Say L, Gülmezoglu AM, Van Look PF. WHO analysis of causes of maternal death: a systematic review. *Lancet* 2006; 367: 1066–74.

2. Brace V, Kernaghan D, Penney G. Learning from adverse clinical outcomes: major obstetric haemorrhage in Scotland, 2003–05. *BJOG* 2007; 114: 1388–96.

3. Centre for Maternal and Child Enquiries. Saving Mothers' Lives: reviewing maternal deaths to make motherhood safer: 2006–08. The Eighth Report in Confidential Enquiries into Maternal Deaths in the United Kingdom. *BJOG* 2011; 118 (Suppl 1): 1–203.

4. Knight M, Kenyon S, Brocklehurst P, Neilson J, Shakespeare J, Kurinczuk JJ (eds) on behalf of MBRRACE UK. *Saving Lives, Improving Mothers' Care: Lessons Learned to Inform Future*

Maternity Care from the UK and Ireland Confidential Enquiries into Maternal Deaths and Morbidity 2009–12. Oxford: National Perinatal Epidemiology Unit, University of Oxford; 2014.

5. Creanga AA, Berg CJ, Syverson C, Seed K, Bruce FC, Callaghan WM. Pregnancy-related mortality in the United States, 2006–2010. *Obstet Gynecol* 2015; 125(1): 5–12.

6. Royal College of Obstetricians and Gynaecologists. *Prevention and Management of Postpartum Haemorrhage.* Green-top Guideline No. 52. London: RCOG; 2009 [www.rcog.org.uk/womens-health/clinical-guidance/prevention-and-management-postpartum-haemorrhage-green-top-52].

7. Lemmens HJ, Bernstein DP, Brodsky JB. Estimating blood volume in obese and morbidly obese patients. *Obes Surg* 2006; 16(6): 773–6.

8. Royal College of Obstetricians and Gynaecologists. *Postpartum Haemorrhage, Prevention and Management.* Green-top Guideline 52. London: RCOG; 2011 [www.rcog.org.uk/womens-health/clinical-guidance/prevention-and-management-postpartum-haemorrhage-green-top-52].

9. Schierhout G, Roberts I. Fluid resuscitation with colloid or crystalloid solutions in critically ill patients: a systematic review of randomised trials. *BMJ* 1998; 316: 961–4.

10. Mittermayr M, Streif W, Haas T, Fries D, Velik-Salchner C, Klingler A, et al. Hemostatic changes after crystalloid or colloid fluid administration during major orthopedic surgery: the role of fibrinogen administration. *Anesth Analg* 2007; 105: 905–17.

11. Shaz BH, Dente CJ, Nicholas J, MacLeod JB, Young AN, Easley K, et al. Increased number of coagulation products in relationship to red blood cell products transfused improves mortality in trauma patients. *Transfusion* 2010; 50: 493–500.

12. James DK, Steer PJ, Weiner CP, Gonik B, Crowther C, Robson S. *High Risk Pregnancy: Management Options*, 4th edn. St Louis: Elsevier; 2010.

13. Royal College Obstetricians and Gynaecologists. *Antepartum Haemorrhage.* Green-top Guideline No. 63. London: RCOG; 2011 [www.rcog.org.uk/womens-health/clinical-guidance/antepartum-haemorrhage-green-top-63].

14. Stones RW, Paterson CM, Saunders NJ. Risk factors for major obstetric haemorrhage. *Eur J Obstet Gynecol Reprod Biol* 1993; 48: 15–18.

15. McDonald S, Prendiville WJ, Elbourne D. Prophylactic ergometriene–oxytocin versus oxytocin for the third stage of labour. *Cochrane Database Syst Rev* 2004; 1: CD000201.

16. Lewis G (ed.) The Confidential Enquiry into Maternal and Child Health (CEMACH). *Saving Mothers' Lives: Reviewing Maternal Deaths to Make Motherhood Safer 2003–2005. The Seventh Report on Confidential Enquiries into Maternal Deaths in the United Kingdom.* London: CEMACH; 2007.

17. Knight M, Kurinczuk JJ, Spark P, Brocklehurst P; United Kingdom Surveillance System Steering Committee. Cesarean delivery and peripartum hysterectomy. *Obstet Gynecol* 2008; 111: 97–105.

18. Lewis G (ed.) The Confidential Enquiry into Maternal and Child Health (CEMACH). *Why Mothers Die 2000–2003. The Sixth Report on Confidential Enquiries into Maternal Deaths in the United Kingdom.* London: RCOG Press; 2004.

19. Gülmezoglu AM, Forna F, Villar J, Hofmeyr GJ. Prostaglandins for prevention of postpartum haemorrhage.*Cochrane Database Syst Rev* 2004; 1: CD000494.

20. Mousa HA, Alfirevic Z. Treatment for primary postpartum haemorrhage. *Cochrane Database Syst Rev* 2007; 1: CD003249.

21. Novikova N, Hofmeyr GJ. Tranexamic acid for preventing postpartum haemorrhage. *Cochrane Database Syst Rev* 2010; 7: CD007872.

22. Shakur H, Elbourne D, Gülmezoglu M, Alfirevic Z, Ronsmans C, Allen E, et al. The WOMAN Trial (World Maternal Antifibrinolytic Trial): tranexamic acid for the treatment of postpartum haemorrhage: an international randomised, double blind placebo controlled trial. *Trials* 2010; 11: 40.

23. Franchini M, Lippi G, Franchi M. The use of recombinant activated factor VII in obstetric and gynaecological haemorrhage. *BJOG* 2007; 114: 8–15.

24. Maier RC. Control of postpartum hemorrhage with uterine packing. *Am J Obstet Gynecol* 1993; 169: 317–21; discussion 321–3.

25. Frenzel D, Condous GS, Papageorghiou AT, McWhinney NA. The use of the "tamponade test" to stop massive obstetric haemorrhage in placenta accreta. *BJOG* 2005; 112: 676–7.

26. National Collaborating Centre for Women's and Children's Health. *Intrapartum Care: Care of Healthy Women and their Babies durng Childbirth*. London: RCOG; 2007.

27. B-Lynch C, Coker A, Lawal AH, Abu J, Cowen MJ. The B-Lynch surgical technique for the control of massive postpartum haemorrhage: an alternative to hysterectomy? Five cases reported. *BJOG* 1997; 104: 372–5.

28. Treloar EJ, Anderson RS, Andrews HS, Bailey JL. Uterine necrosis following B-Lynch suture for primary postpartum haemorrhage. *BJOG* 2006; 113: 486–8.

29. Pechtor K, Richards B, Paterson H. Antenatal catastrophic uterine rupture at 32 weeks of gestation after previous B-Lynch suture. *BJOG* 2010; 117: 889–91.

30. Bateman BT, Mhyre JM, Callaghan WM, et al. Peripartum hysterectomy in the United States: nationwide 14 year experience. *Am J Obstet Gynecol* 2012; 206: 63.e1–8.

Module 9
Shoulder dystocia

Key learning points

- Shoulder dystocia is unpredictable.
- Understand that only progressively increasing axial traction be applied until reaching resistance and never exceeding that used for a routine vaginal delivery.
- Understand maneuvers required to release shoulders during a shoulder dystocia.
- Understand the importance of clear and accurate documentation.
- Be aware of the potential complications of shoulder dystocia.

Common difficulties observed in training drills

- Failing to state the problem.
- Not calling for the neonatologist.
- Inability to gain appropriate vaginal access.
- Confusion over the difference between axial, downward, and lateral traction.
- Confusion over internal rotational maneuvers.
- Resorting to excessive traction to effect delivery.
- Use of fundal pressure.

Introduction

Definition

Shoulder dystocia has many definitions but it is perhaps easiest to define it as whenever additional maneuvers (such as McRoberts' position and suprapubic

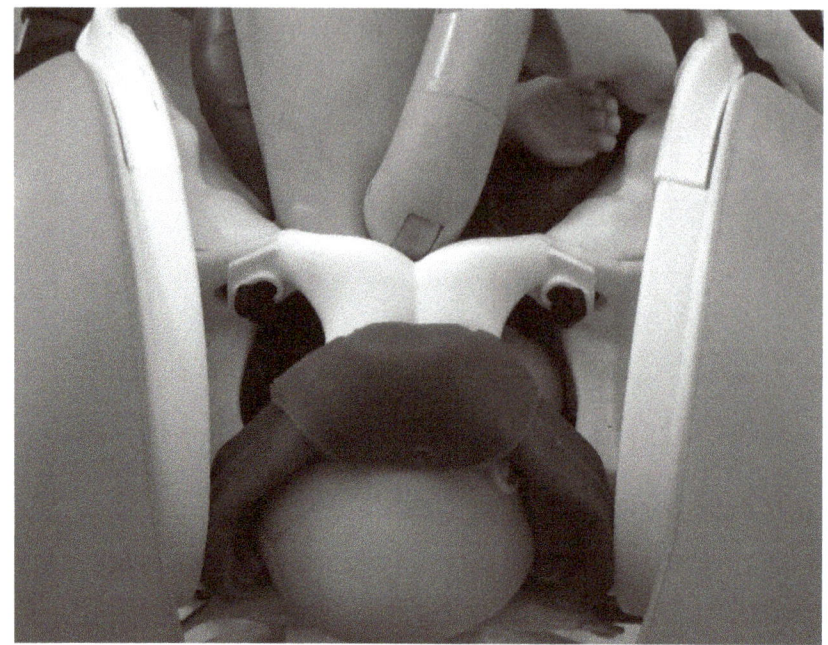

Figure 9.1 Shoulder dystocia with anterior fetal shoulder impacted on maternal symphysis pubis

pressure) are required to complete delivery after progressively applied axial traction has failed to release the shoulders.[1]

Incidence

There is wide variation in the reported incidence of shoulder dystocia due in part to differences in definition.[2] Studies involving the largest number of vaginal deliveries report an incidence between 0.58% and 0.70%.[3,4,5,6,7,8]

Pathophysiology

When a shoulder dystocia occurs, it is usually the anterior fetal shoulder that impacts on the maternal symphysis pubis following delivery of the head, preventing delivery of the body (Figure 9.1). Less commonly, the posterior fetal shoulder impacts on the maternal sacral promontory.

Risk factors for shoulder dystocia

A number of antenatal and intrapartum characteristics are reported to be associated with shoulder dystocia (Box 9.1), but even a combination of risk factors is poorly predictive.[9,10] Only about one in six cases of shoulder dystocia that result in neonatal morbidity are predicted by conventional risk factors.[11]

Box 9.1 Risk factors for shoulder dystocia

Prelabor	Intrapartum
Prior shoulder dystocia	Prolonged 1st stage
Macrosomia	Prolonged 2nd stage
Maternal diabetes mellitus	Labor augmentation
Maternal obesity	Vacuum assisted vaginal delivery

A prior shoulder dystocia is a risk factor for recurrent shoulder dystocia. The rate of shoulder dystocia in women who experienced a shoulder dystocia during a prior delivery is estimated to be 10 times higher than the general population.[12] This may, however, be an underestimate, as cesarean deliveries are common after severe shoulder dystocia.

Macrosomia

The greater the fetal birth weight, the higher the risk of shoulder dystocia. One review of 14,721 births reported the rates of shoulder dystocia in non-diabetic mothers was 1% in infants weighing less than 4,000 g, 10% in infants weighing 4,000 to 4,499 g, and 23% in infants weighing more than 4,500 g.[13] However, macrosomia remains a weak predictor of shoulder dystocia. A large majority of infants with a birth weight of greater than 4,500 g do not develop shoulder dystocia and up to 50% of cases of shoulder dystocia occur in infants with a birth weight less than 4,000 g.[4] Furthermore, antenatal detection of macrosomia is poor: third-trimester ultrasound scans have at least a 10% margin of error for actual birth weight and detect only 60% of infants weighing over 4,500 g.[14]

Maternal diabetes mellitus

Maternal diabetes mellitus increases the risk of shoulder dystocia.[9] Infants of diabetic mothers have a two- to four-fold increased risk of shoulder dystocia compared with infants of the same birth weight born to non-diabetic mothers.[9,15] The increased risk is attributed to a difference in body proportions of babies born to diabetic mothers.

Instrumental delivery

There is a higher rate of shoulder dystocia associated with vacuum assisted delivery and emergency mid forceps delivery compared to a spontaneous vaginal delivery;[16] in contrast a low/outlet forceps delivery may well lower the shoulder dystocia rate.[17]

Obesity

Women with a raised body mass index (BMI) are at higher risk of shoulder dystocia than women with a normal BMI.[18] However, women who are obese tend to have larger babies and the association between maternal obesity and shoulder dystocia may well be more attributable to fetal macrosomia rather than the maternal obesity itself.[19]

Key points

- The majority of shoulder dystocia cases occur in women with no risk factors.
- Shoulder dystocia is an unpredictable and therefore a largely unpreventable event.
- While clinicians should be aware of existing risk factors, they must always be alert to the possibility of shoulder dystocia with any delivery.

Prevention

Shoulder dystocia can only be prevented by cesarean section. Yet even with suspected fetal macrosomia, elective cesarean section does not lower the injury rate,[20] and is not recommended as a method of reducing potential morbidity from possible shoulder dystocia. It has been estimated that an additional 2,345 cesarean deliveries would be required to prevent one permanent brachial plexus injury from shoulder dystocia.[14]

Elective cesarean section is recommended for women with diabetes and suspected fetal macrosomia (>4.5 kg) or where the estimated fetal weight is greater than 5 kg in a woman without diabetes.[21] This is because of the higher incidence of shoulder dystocia and brachial plexus injury in these subgroups.

Management

There are numerous maneuvers that can be used to resolve shoulder dystocia. Forces applied to the fetus during delivery are a combination of the maternal (uterine plus valsalva) and accoucheur efforts to overcome birth canal resistance.

An effective algorithm for the management of shoulder dystocia is shown in Figure 9.2.

There is no evidence that any one intervention is superior to another; therefore it makes sense that algorithms begin with the least invasive maneuvers, progressing through to maneuvers that are more invasive. Variations in the sequence of actions may be appropriate.

Recognition of shoulder dystocia

- There may be difficulty with delivery of the face and chin.
- After the head is born, it remains tightly applied to the vulva.
- The chin retracts and depresses the perineum – the "turtle-neck" sign.
- The anterior shoulder fails to release with maternal pushing and/or when progressive and no more than routine axial traction is applied.

Call for help

- Use the emergency alarm (not the call bell).
- Call for:
  - ☐ the most experienced labor nurse on the floor
  - ☐ additional nursing staff
  - ☐ the most experienced obstetrician available
  - ☐ neonatologist (often forgotten).
- Consider calling the anesthesiologist.

Clearly state the problem. State that there is a "shoulder dystocia" as help arrives.

Note the time the head was delivered (start the timer or mark the EFM, if monitoring).

Ask the mother to stop pushing. Pushing should be discouraged, as it will not resolve the dystocia and may increase the severity and therefore the risk of neurological and orthopedic complications.

McRoberts' maneuver

The McRoberts' maneuver is considered an effective intervention.[19] It has a low rate of complication and is one of the least invasive maneuvers, and is commonly employed first.

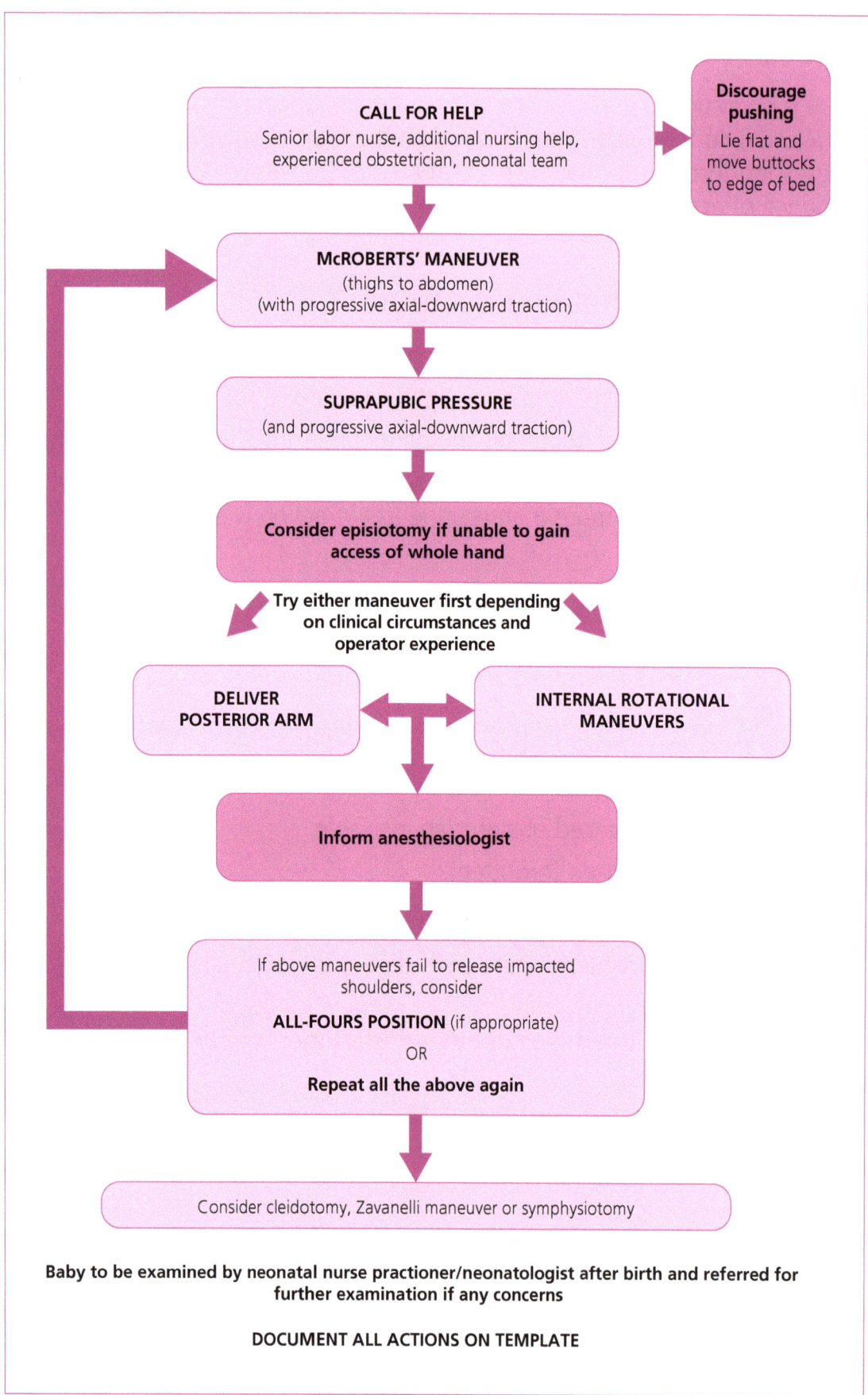

Figure 9.2 Algorithm for the management of shoulder dystocia

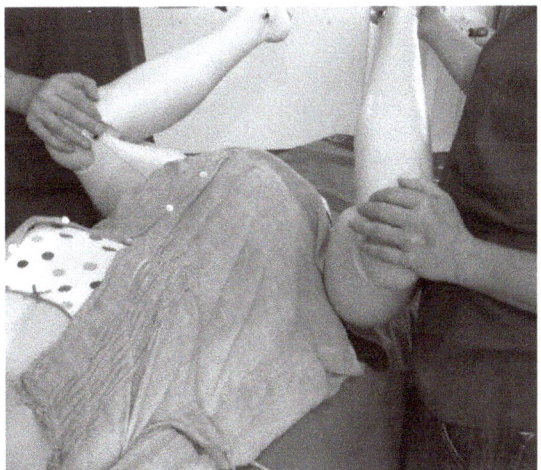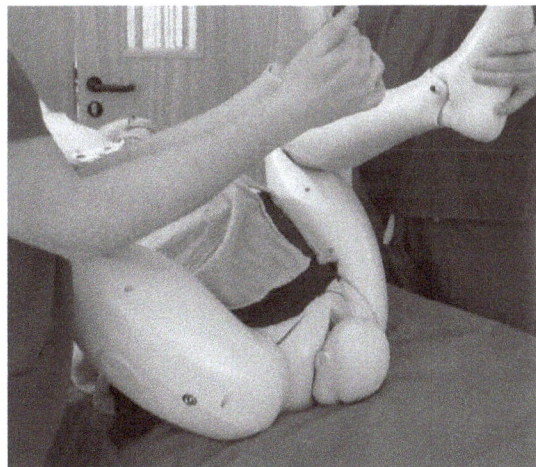

Figure 9.3 McRoberts' position

Lie the mother flat and remove any pillows from under her back. Bring her to the end of the bed and/or remove the end of the bed to make vaginal access easier. With one assistant on either side, hyperflex the mother's legs against her abdomen so that her knees are up towards her ears (Figure 9.3). If the mother is in the lithotomy position, her legs will need to be removed from the supports to achieve McRoberts' positioning.

The McRoberts' position acts to relieve the obstruction through at least two very different mechanisms. Firstly, it increases the relative anteroposterior diameter of the pelvic inlet by rotating the maternal pelvis cephalic and straightening the sacrum relative to the lumbar spine. Secondly, it increases the transfer of the maternal valsalva force to the uterine, actually doubling the total force brought to bear on the fetus from above.[22] Therefore McRoberts' does not mean an easier delivery; it means the accoucheur needs to use less force since the mother's contribution has increased. Though successful in relieving impaction, its use has in some reports actually been associated with an increasing rate of brachial plexus injury.[35] McRoberts' position prophylactically before delivery of the head in anticipation of shoulder dystocia is ineffective; therefore prophylactic McRoberts' is not recommended.

Progressive axial traction

Traditional experiential training holds that the same degree of traction as applied during a normal birth and in an axial direction, i.e. in line with the axis of the fetal spine (Figure 9.4), should then be applied to the baby's head to assess whether the shoulders have been released. *We suggest applying progressively increasing axial traction until reaching resistance and never exceeding that used for a routine vaginal delivery. That way, only the minimal*

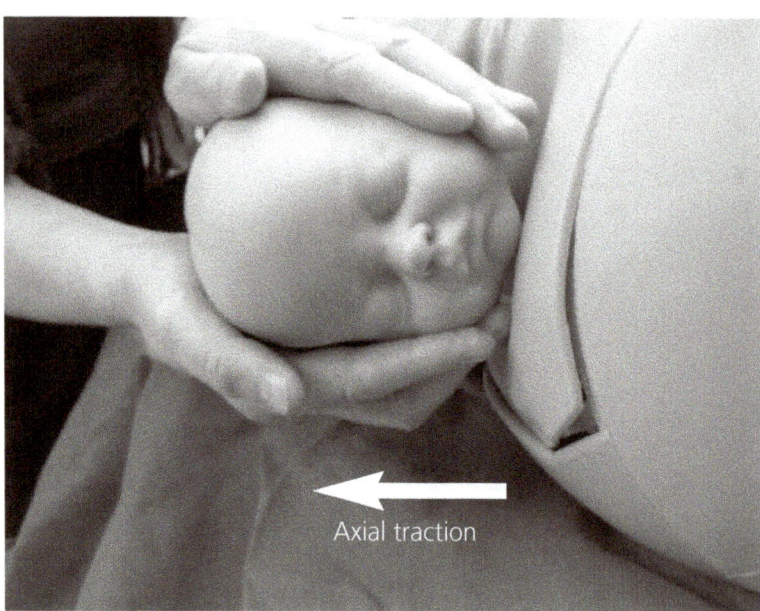

Axial traction

Figure 9.4 Axial traction

amount of force required for an individual delivery will be applied. With the axial traction, the accoucheur moves their hands (and the baby's head) toward but parallel to the floor (never moving the baby's head lateral). If the anterior shoulder is not released with McRoberts' position, move on to the next maneuver. Do not continue to apply traction to the baby's head if the obstruction has not been relieved.

> **Remember: shoulder dystocia is a "bony problem" where the baby's shoulder is obstructed by the mother's pelvis. If the entrapment is not released by McRoberts' position, another release maneuver, and not traction, is required to free the shoulder and complete the delivery.**

Suprapubic pressure

The application of suprapubic pressure seeks to reduce the fetal bisacromial (shoulder-to-shoulder) diameter and rotate the anterior fetal shoulder into the wider oblique diameter of the pelvis. The anterior shoulder is freed to slip underneath the symphysis pubis with progressive axial traction as described above.[23]

An assistant should apply suprapubic pressure from the side of the fetal back (in the direction the fetal face is watching) using a clasped hand position

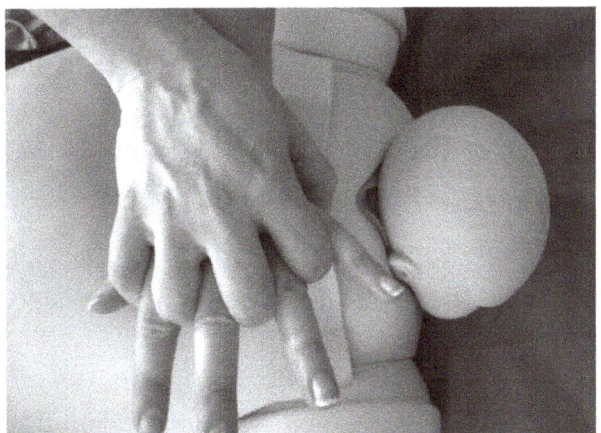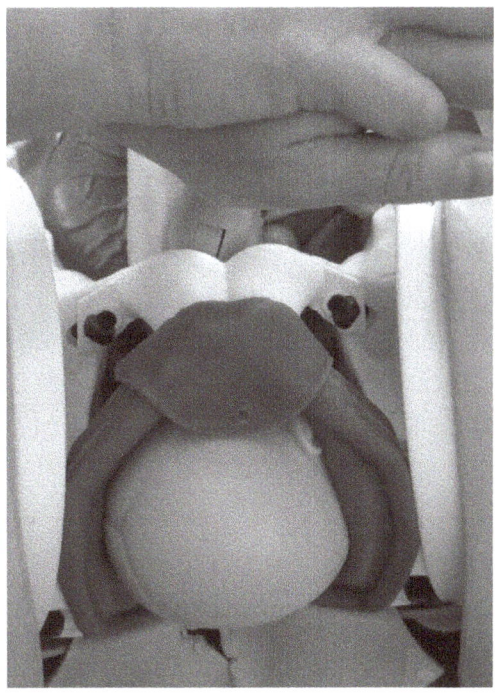

Figure 9.5 Applying suprapubic pressure

similar to that used for CPR. Pressure is applied in a downward and lateral direction, just above the maternal symphysis pubis, to push the posterior portion of the anterior shoulder towards the fetal chest (Figure 9.5). If you are unsure of the location of the fetal back, suprapubic pressure should be applied from the most likely side of the fetal back and, if this is unsuccessful at resolving the dystocia, suprapubic pressure can be attempted from the other side.

There is no evidence that suprapubic pressure applied in a pulsating movement is any better than continuous suprapubic pressure or that it should be performed for 30 seconds for it to be effective. Only progressive axial traction as described above up to the degree used for a routine delivery should be applied to the fetal head when assessing whether the maneuver has been successful. Again, if the anterior shoulder is not released with suprapubic pressure and progressive axial traction as previously described, the next maneuver should be attempted.

Evaluate the need for an episiotomy

Often the perineum has torn or an episiotomy cut before delivery of the head. Cutting an episiotomy after delivery of the head will not relieve the bony obstruction of shoulder dystocia. There is almost always enough room to gain internal access with the correct technique without performing an episiotomy.[24] On rare occasions, cutting an episiotomy allows the accoucheur more space to facilitate internal vaginal maneuvers (delivery of the posterior arm or internal rotation of the shoulders).

Internal maneuvers

There are two categories of internal vaginal maneuver that can be performed should McRoberts' position and suprapubic pressure not be effective: delivery of the posterior arm and internal rotational maneuvers. There are no randomized trials suggesting one is superior to the other. There are, however, case series suggesting the rate of brachial plexus injury is lower with delivery of the posterior arm.[25,26] All internal maneuvers start with the same action: inserting the whole hand posteriorly into the sacral hollow.

Gaining internal vaginal access

When shoulder dystocia occurs, the problem is usually that the anterior shoulder is trapped above the symphysis pubis. There is a temptation to try to gain vaginal access anteriorly so as to perform maneuvers. However, there is no room to execute any useful release maneuvers underneath the pubic arch (Figure 9.6).

Vaginal access can be gained most easily posteriorly into the sacral hollow, which is the most spacious part of the pelvis. The accoucheur should scrunch up their hand (as if putting on a tight bracelet), to facilitate accurate placement to deliver the posterior arm or perform internal rotation (Figure 9.7).

Delivery of the posterior arm

Delivering the posterior arm reduces the diameter of the fetal body by the width of the arm, which often provides sufficient room to resolve the shoulder dystocia.

Fetuses often lie with their arms flexed across their chest and so as your hand enters the vagina posteriorly, you will feel the fetal hand and forearm of the posterior arm (Figure 9.8). It is easiest if you insert the hand on the side the fetus is facing. Take hold of the fetal wrist (with your fingers and thumb) and gently deliver the posterior arm in a straight line (Figure 9.9). This movement of the fetal arm is similar to the action of "putting your hand up in class." Once the posterior arm is delivered (Figure 9.10), apply progressive axial traction to the fetal head as described earlier. If the shoulder dystocia has resolved, the baby should deliver relatively easily.

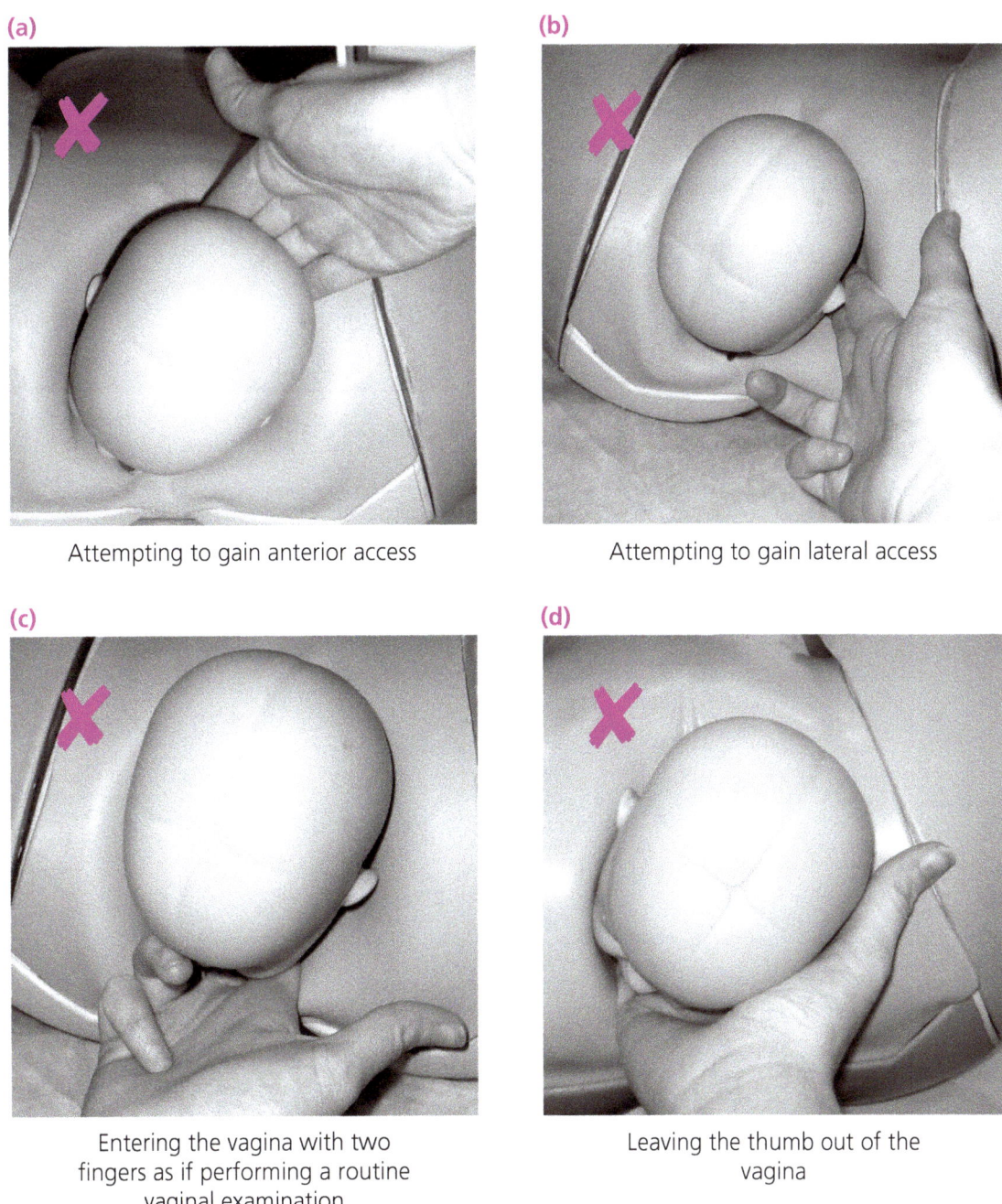

(a)

Attempting to gain anterior access

(b)

Attempting to gain lateral access

(c)

Entering the vagina with two
fingers as if performing a routine
vaginal examination

(d)

Leaving the thumb out of the
vagina

Figure 9.6 Incorrect attempts at gaining vaginal access

If, despite delivering the posterior arm, the shoulder dystocia has not resolved, support the head and posterior arm and gently rotate the baby through 180 degrees. The posterior shoulder will then become the new anterior shoulder and should be below the symphysis pubis, thereby resolving the dystocia. However, this is very rarely required.

It is a much more difficult to deliver a posterior arm that is extended straight against the body, rather than flexed. The arm can sometimes be flexed so that

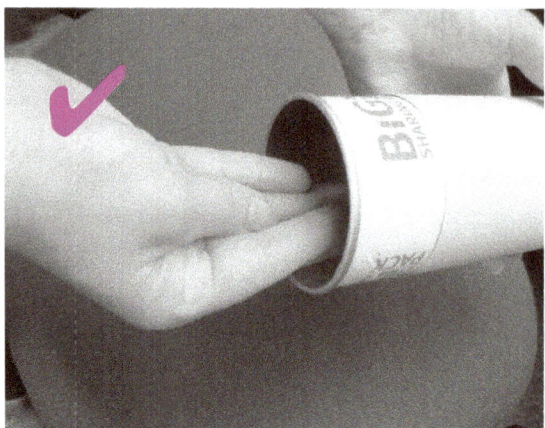 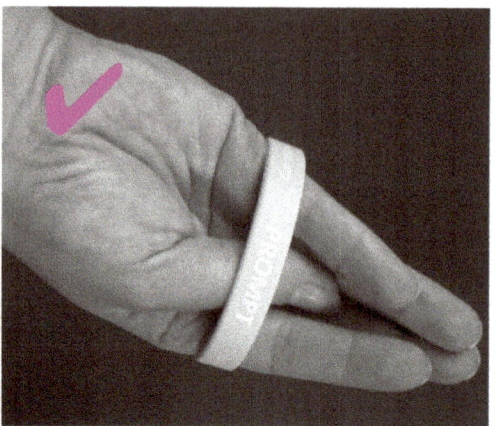

Figure 9.7 Correct vaginal access

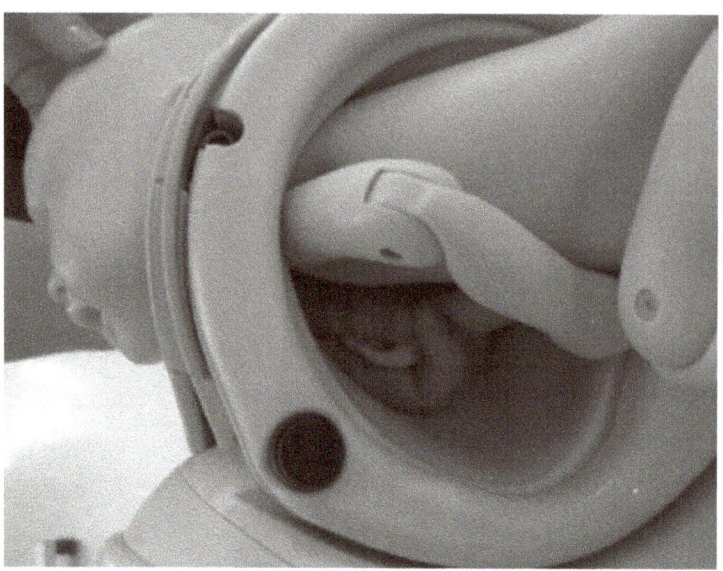

Figure 9.8 Location of the posterior arm

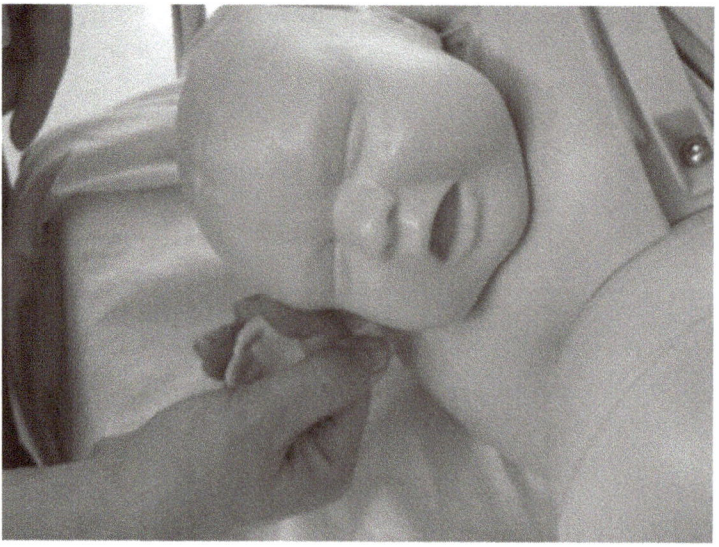

Figure 9.9 Delivery of the posterior arm in a straight line

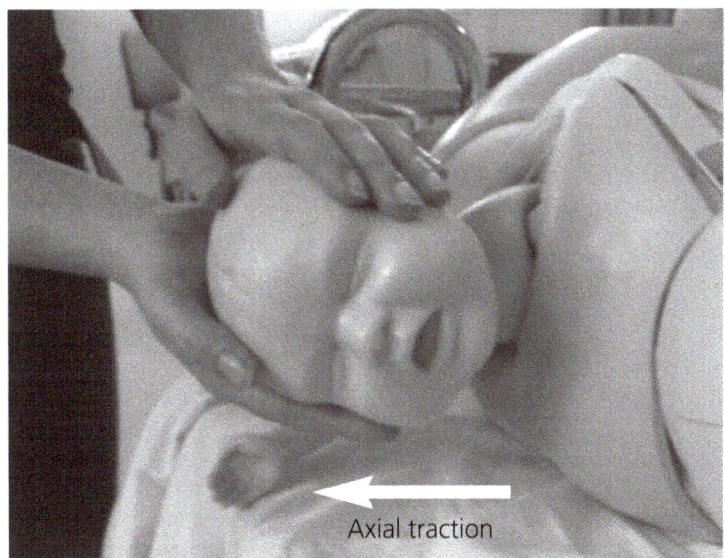

Axial traction

Figure 9.10 Axial traction to deliver the rest of the body

the wrist can be grasped using pressure in the antecubital fossa followed by pressure with fingers to the back of the forearm just below the elbow. This should flex the posterior arm. The wrist can then be grasped and the arm delivered as previously described. *Do not pull on the upper arm if you cannot reach the wrist, as this can cause a humeral fracture.*

Remember to ask that suprapubic pressure be stopped while you gain internal vaginal access and attempt internal maneuvers.

Internal rotational maneuvers

The aims of internal rotation are:

- to move the fetal shoulders (the bisacromial diameter) out of the narrowest diameter of the maternal pelvis (the anterior–posterior) and into a wider pelvic diameter (the oblique or transverse)
- to use the maternal pelvic anatomy – as the fetal shoulders are rotated within the maternal pelvis, the fetal shoulder descends through the pelvis owing to the bony architecture of the pelvis.

Originally described independently by Woods and Rubin, rotation can be most easily achieved by pressing on the anterior (front) or posterior (back) aspect of the posterior (lowermost) shoulder (Figure 9.11). Pressure on the posterior aspect of the posterior shoulder has the added benefit of reducing the shoulder diameter by adducting the shoulders (scrunching the shoulders inwards). Rotation should move the shoulders into the wider oblique diameter, resolving the shoulder dystocia, so that delivery is possible with progressive

(a) (b)

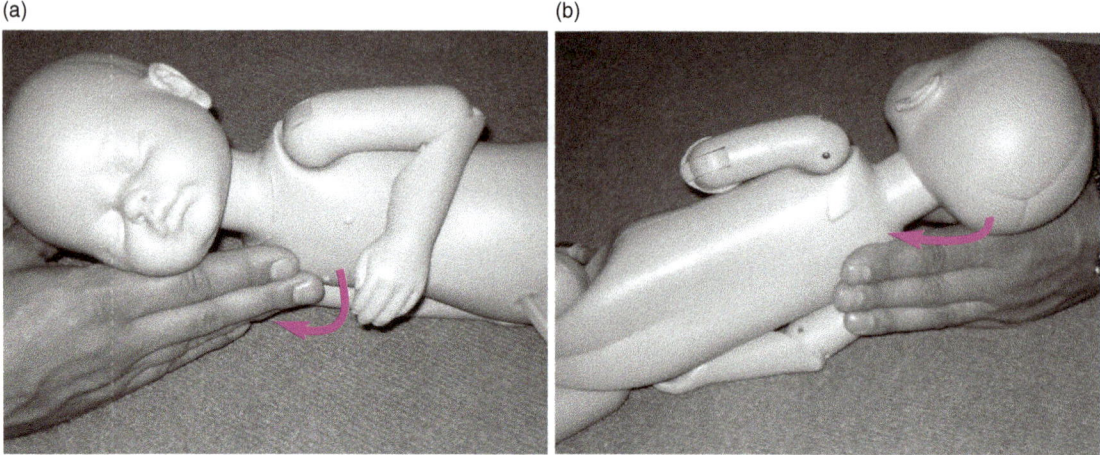

Figure 9.11 Internal rotational maneuvers: (a) pressure on the anterior aspect of the posterior shoulder to achieve rotation; (b) pressure on the posterior aspect of the posterior shoulder to achieve rotation

axial traction as previously described. If delivery does not occur, continue the pressure and, by swapping hands, rotate the shoulders a complete turn (180-degree rotation). This maneuver (as with rotation after delivery of the posterior arm) substitutes the anterior shoulder for the posterior shoulder and should resolve the dystocia.

If pressure in one direction has no effect, try to rotate the shoulders in the opposite direction by pressing on the other side of the fetal posterior shoulder (that is, change from pressing on the front of the baby's shoulder to the back of the baby's shoulder or vice versa). If you are struggling, try changing the hand you are using.

If pressure on the posterior shoulder is unsuccessful, apply pressure on the anterior fetal shoulder. This is more difficult, as it is hard to reach the anterior shoulder. From the sacral hollow, follow the fetal back up to the anterior shoulder. Apply pressure on the posterior aspect of the anterior shoulder to adduct and rotate the shoulders into the oblique diameter.

While attempting to rotate the fetal shoulders from the inside of the pelvis, you can instruct a colleague to perform suprapubic pressure to assist your rotation. Ensure that you are pushing with and not against each other.

While there is no comparative evidence to select one maneuver over another, it is clear that the risk of a brachial plexus injury increases with the number of maneuvers performed to relieve the obstruction. There are likely multiple explanations for this observation, all offset by using a definitive maneuver and using progressive axial traction as described previously so that only the minimal force for that individual delivery is used.

All-fours position

The all-fours position has been described to have an 83% success rate in one small case series.[27] Individual circumstances should guide the accoucheur's decision whether to try the all-fours technique before or after attempting internal rotation and delivery of the posterior arm. For a slim mobile woman without epidural anesthesia and with a single attendant, the all-fours position is less invasive and thus probably more appropriate. For a less mobile woman with epidural anesthesia in place, internal maneuvers may be more appropriate.

Roll the mother on to her hands and knees so that the maternal weight lies evenly on them. This simple change of position may dislodge the anterior shoulder and the woman may spontaneously push, or progressive axial traction may be applied to the fetal head as previously described, to ascertain if the dystocia has been resolved. If dystocia remains, the all-fours position also facilitates access to the posterior shoulder to enable internal maneuvers to be performed.

> **Remember when the woman is in an all-fours position that the maternal sacral hollow and the fetal posterior shoulder will both be uppermost.**

Additional maneuvers

Several salvage maneuvers have been described for those cases resistant to all standard maneuvers; however, their use is very rare if the standard maneuvers are performed correctly.

Vaginal replacement of the head (Zavanelli maneuver) followed by cesarean delivery has been described with variable success.[28,29,30] While the maternal safety of this procedure is unknown, it is often traumatic for the fetus; and a high proportion of fetuses may have irreversible hypoxia–acidosis by this stage. As the uterus will have contracted following delivery of the fetal head, a tocolytic (e.g., terbutaline 250 mcg subcutaneously or sublingual glyceryl trinitrate) should be given prior to any attempts to replace the fetal head to reduce the risk of uterine rupture.

Symphysiotomy (partial surgical division of the maternal symphysis pubis ligament) has been suggested as a potentially useful procedure. However, it is rarely taught in the industrialized world and there is a high incidence of serious maternal morbidity and poor neonatal outcome.[31] Other techniques, including the use of a posterior axillary sling, have been reported but there are few data available.[32,33]

How much time do I have?

The condition of the baby at delivery is dependent on the head-to-body interval but also the fetal condition at the start of the dystocia. However, it is not possible to recommend an absolute time limit for the management of shoulder dystocia, as the head-to-body birth interval that each individual fetus can withstand without hypoxia occurring will vary with individual clinical circumstances. Often, but not always, the umbilical cord is occluded.

One review of fatal cases of shoulder dystocia noted that 47% of the babies that died did so within 5 minutes of the head being delivered; however, a very high proportion of cases had grossly abnormal EFM patterns prior to delivery of the head.[34] A more recent review concluded there was a very low rate of hypoxic ischemic injury if the head-to-body delivery time was less than 5 minutes.[35] Imposing time limits may cause accoucheurs to resort to more forceful traction as the 5-minute time limit approaches, suggesting it is better to emphasize the importance of managing the problem as efficiently as possible to avoid hypoxia and as carefully as possible to avoid unnecessary trauma.

What to avoid

Traction

It may be an instinctive reaction to pull on the fetal head in an attempt to deliver the baby. However, traction alone will not resolve the dystocia and **excessive traction (more than necessary) must be avoided**.

In addition, traction applied so that the fetal head moves lateral (or described incorrectly by some as downward) toward its shoulder (in contrast to axial traction) is strongly associated with brachial plexus injury. Therefore **lateral traction on the fetal head** must be avoided in all deliveries.

There is also evidence that traction applied quickly with momentum, such as a tug or "jerk" rather than traction applied progressively but not exceeding routine may be more damaging to the brachial plexus[36] (imagine trying to snap a piece of cotton – it is much easier to break it with a quick pull than a slow one).

> **Progressive axial downward traction should always be applied slowly and gently and not with sudden force or in a downward lateral direction.**

Fundal pressure

Fundal pressure is associated with an increased rate of brachial plexus injury and rupture of the uterus. It should **not be applied** during shoulder dystocia.[29]

Documentation

Accurate documentation of a difficult and potentially traumatic delivery is essential. It is important to write a clear explanation of the maneuvers performed (it is not essential to use names of maneuvers) such that someone else reading later can reproduce those actions. It may be helpful to use a template to aid accurate record keeping. An example is provided in Figure 9.12.

It is important to record:

- the time of delivery of the head
- the anterior fetal shoulder at the time of the dystocia (right or left)
- the maneuvers performed, their sequence, and times
- the traction applied – progressive axial as described earlier keeping the baby's head parallel to the floor
- the time the body was delivered
- the staff in attendance and the time they arrived
- the condition of the baby
- umbilical cord blood acid–base measurements.

Parents

Shoulder dystocia is a frightening and potentially traumatic experience for the mother and her attending family. It is important to tell the parents what is happening and to give the mother clear instructions during the emergency. Both the delivery and the reason for the use of maneuvers should be discussed after delivery.

A neonatologist should immediately review any baby with a suspected injury following shoulder dystocia. A woman who has had a prior delivery complicated by shoulder dystocia should be referred to a perinatologist antenatal unit in subsequent pregnancies to discuss antenatal care and mode of birth.

| SHOULDER DYSTOCIA DOCUMENTATION | | | | | PROMPT Making Childbirth Safer, Together |

Date .... Time ....

Person completing form.......................Designation...........

Signature ....

Mother's Name :
Date of birth :
Hospital Number
Physician

Called for help at:

Staff present at delivery of head:		Additional staff attending for delivery of shoulders		
Name	Role	Name	Role	Time arrived

Procedures used to assist delivery	By whom	Time	Order	Details	Reason if not performed
McRoberts' position:					
Suprapubic pressure:				From maternal left / right (circle as appropriate)	
Episiotomy:				Not required as enough room for access / perineal tear present / already performed for delivery of head (circle as appropriate)	
Delivery of posterior arm:				**Right** / **left** arm (circle as appropriate)	
Internal rotational maneuvers:					
Description of rotation:					
Description of traction:	Routine axial (as in normal vaginal birth)	Other -		Reason if not routine	
Other maneuvers used:					

Mode of delivery of head:	Spontaneous		Instrumental – vacuum / forceps	
Time of delivery of head:	Time of delivery of baby		Head-to-body delivery interval	
Fetal position during dystocia:	Head facing maternal **left** **Left** fetal shoulder anterior		Head facing maternal **right** **Right** fetal shoulder anterior	
Birth weight kg	Apgar	1 min :	5 mins :	10 mins :
Cord gases:	Art pH:	Art BE:	Venous pH :	Venous BE :
Explanation to parents	Yes	By		

Neonatologist called: Yes / No   Time arrived: ....   Neonatologist's name : ....

Baby assessment at delivery Any sign of arm weakness? Any sign of potential bony fracture? Baby admitted to Neonatal Intensive Care Unit? Assessment by	Yes Yes Yes	No No No	If yes to any of these questions for review and follow up by neonatologist

Modified from North Bristol NHS Trust.

Figure 9.12 An example of a shoulder dystocia documentation template

Consequences of shoulder dystocia

Shoulder dystocia has a high perinatal morbidity and mortality rate.[5] Maternal morbidity is also increased (Box 9.2).

Acidosis

Shoulder dystocia is an acute life-threatening event. A healthy fetus can compensate during shoulder dystocia for only a finite amount of time. Babies born with a severe metabolic acidosis may develop hypoxic ischemic encephalopathy (HIE), with or without long-term neurological damage. The necessary resuscitation equipment should be prepared and neonatal staff called as soon as shoulder dystocia is diagnosed in case neonatal resuscitation is required.

Brachial plexus injury

Brachial plexus injury is one of the most important complications of shoulder dystocia and it affects approximately 1 in 2,300 deliveries.[37] Though shoulder dystocia is not preventable, permanent brachial plexus injury may be.[38] The primary mechanism for brachial plexus injury is thought to be lateral traction on the fetal head during shoulder dystocia, although other mechanisms of injury have been proposed. Brachial plexus injuries may be a complication of normal labor and are reported after cesarean section. Injuries can be divided into upper (Erb's palsy), lower (Klumpke's palsy), or total brachial plexus injury:

- **Erb's palsy** is the most common injury. The upper arm is flaccid and the lower arm is extended and rotated towards the body with the hand held in a classic "waiter's tip" posture. Up to 90% of Erb's palsies recover by 12 months.

Box 9.2 Perinatal morbidity and mortality	
Perinatal	**Maternal**
Stillbirth	Postpartum hemorrhage
Hypoxia	Third- and fourth-degree tears
Brachial plexus injury	Uterine rupture
Fractures (humeral and clavicular)	Psychological distress

- **Klumpke's palsy** is less common. The hand is limp, with no movement of the fingers. The recovery rate is lower and only around 40% of injuries resolve by 12 months.

- **Total brachial plexus** injury occurs in approximately 20% of brachial plexus injuries. There is complete sensory and motor deficit of the entire arm, rendering it completely paralyzed without sensation. Horner syndrome may also be present, caused by injury to the sympathetic nerve that results in contraction of the pupil and ptosis of the eyelid on the affected side. Full functional recovery is rare without surgical intervention. The prognosis is worse if Horner syndrome is present.

Humeral and clavicular fractures

Humeral and clavicular fractures may also occur during shoulder dystocia. These fractures usually heal quickly and have a good prognosis.

Shoulder dystocia is an unpredictable obstetric emergency	
Problem	Clearly state the problem
Pediatricians	Immediately call the pediatrician/neonatologist
Position	McRoberts' or all fours
Pressure	Suprapubic (NOT FUNDAL) pressure
Posterior	Vaginal access gained posteriorly
Perineum	Get the whole hand in
Pull	Don't keep pulling if a maneuver has not worked
Protocol	Documentation should be clear and concise
Parents	Communication and explanation are essential

References

1. Resnick R. Management of shoulder girdle dystocia. *Clin Obstet Gynecol* 1980; 23: 559–64.

2. Gherman RB. Shoulder dystocia: an evidence-based evaluation of the obstetric nightmare. *Clin Obstet Gynecol* 2002; 45: 345–62.

3. McFarland M, Hod M, Piper JM, Xenakis EM, Langer O. Are labor abnormalities more common in shoulder dystocia? *Am J Obstet Gynecol* 1995; 173: 1211–14.

4. Baskett TF, Allen AC. Perinatal implications of shoulder dystocia. *Obstet Gynecol* 1995; 86: 14–17.

5. Gherman RB, Ouzounian JG, Goodwin TM. Obstetric maneuvers for shoulder dystocia and associated fetal morbidity. *Am J Obstet Gynecol* 1998; 178: 1126–30.

6. McFarland MB, Langer O, Piper JM, Berkus MD. Perinatal outcome and the type and number of maneuvers in shoulder dystocia. *Int J Gynaecol Obstet* 1996; 55: 219–24.

7. Ouzounian JG, Gherman RB. Shoulder dystocia: are historic risk factors reliable predictors? *Am J Obstet Gynecol* 2005; 192: 1933–5.

8. Smith RB, Lane C, Pearson JF. Shoulder dystocia: what happens at the next delivery? *Br J Obstet Gynaecol* 1994; 101: 713–15.

9. Nesbitt TS, Gilbert WM, Herrchen B. Shoulder dystocia and associated risk factors with macrosomic infants born in California. *Am J Obstet Gynecol* 1998; 179: 476–80.

10. Bahar AM. Risk factors and fetal outcome in cases of shoulder dystocia compared with normal deliveries of a similar birthweight. *Br J Obstet Gynaecol* 1996; 103: 868–72.

11. Gross TL, Sokol RJ, Williams T, Thompson K. Shoulder dystocia: a fetal–physician risk. *Am J Obstet Gynecol* 1987; 156: 1408–18.

12. Mehta SH, Blackwell SC, Chadha R, Sokol RJ. Shoulder dystocia and the next delivery: outcomes and management. *J Matern Fetal Neonatal Med* 2007; 20: 729–33.

13. Acker DB, Sachs BP, Friedman EA. Risk factors for shoulder dystocia in the average-weight infant. *Obstet Gynecol* 1986; 67: 614–18.

14. Rouse DJ, Owen J. Prophylactic cesarean delivery for fetal macrosomia diagnosed by means of ultrasonography: A Faustian bargain? *Am J Obstet Gynecol* 1999; 181: 332–8.

15. Acker DB, Sachs BP, Friedman EA. Risk factors for shoulder dystocia. *Obstet Gynecol* 1985; 66: 762–8.

16. Benedetti TJ, Gabbe SG. Shoulder dystocia. A complication of fetal macrosomia and prolonged second stage of labor with midpelvic delivery. *Obstet Gynecol* 1978; 52: 526–9.

17. Caughey AB, Sandberg PL, Zlatnik MG, Thiet MP, Parer JT, Laros RK Jr. Forceps compared with vacuum: rates of neonatal and maternal morbidity. *Obstet Gynecol* 2005; 106: 908–12.

18. Sandmire HF, O'Halloin TJ. Shoulder dystocia: its incidence and associated risk factors. *Int J Gynaecol Obstet* 1988; 26: 65–73.

19. Usha Kiran TS, Hemmadi S, Bethel J, Evans J. Outcome of pregnancy in a woman with an increased body mass index. *BJOG* 2005; 112: 768–72.

20. Weiner Z, Ben-Shlomo I, Beck-Fruchter R, Goldberg Y, Shalev E. Clinical and ultrasonographic weight estimation in large for gestational age fetus. *Eur J Obstet Gynecol Reprod Biol* 2002; 105(1): 204.

21. Royal College of Obstetricians and Gynaecologists. *Shoulder Dystocia*. Green-top Guideline No. 42. London: RCOG; 2011 [www.rcog.org.uk/womens-health/clinical-guidance/shoulder-dystocia-green-top-42].

22. Buhimschi CS, Buhimschi IA, Malinow A, Weiner CP. Use of McRoberts' position during delivery and increase in pushing efficiency. *Lancet* 2001; 358: 470–1.

23. Lurie S, Ben-Arie A, Hagay Z. The ABC of shoulder dystocia management. *Asia Oceania J Obstet Gynaecol* 1994; 20: 195–7.

24. Hinshaw K. Shoulder dystocia. In Johanson R, Cox C, Grady K, Howell C (eds). *Managing Obstetric Emergencies and Trauma. The MOET Course Manual*. London: RCOG Press; 2003: pp. 165–74.

25. Adler JB, Patterson RL Jr. Erb's palsy. Long-term results of treatment in eighty-eight cases. *J Bone Joint Surg Am* 1967; 49: 1052–64.

26. Baskett TF, Allen AC. Perinatal implications of shoulder dystocia. *Obstet Gynecol* 1995; 86: 14–17.

27. Bruner JP, Drummond SB, Meenan AL, Gaskin IM. All-fours maneuver for reducing shoulder dystocia during labor. *J Reprod Med* 1998; 43: 439–43.

28. Sandberg EC. The Zavanelli maneuver: a potentially revolutionary method for the resolution of shoulder dystocia. *Am J Obstet Gynecol* 1985; 152: 479–84.

29. Vaithilingam N, Davies D. Cephalic replacement for shoulder dystocia: three cases. *BJOG* 2005; 112: 674–5.

30. Spellacy WN. The Zavanelli maneuver for fetal shoulder dystocia. Three cases with poor outcomes. *J Reprod Med* 1995; 40: 543–4.

31. Goodwin TM, Banks E, Millar LK, Phelan JP. Catastrophic shoulder dystocia and emergency symphysiotomy. *Am J Obstet Gynecol* 1997; 177: 463–4.

32. Gherman R. Posterior axillary sling traction: another empiric technique for shoulder dystocia alleviation? *Obstet Gynecol* 2009; 113: 478–9.

33. Hofmeyr GJ, Cluver CA. Posterior axilla sling traction for intractable shoulder dystocia. *BJOG* 2009; 116: 1818–20.

34. Maternal and Child Health Research Consortium. *Confidential Enquiry into Stillbirths and Deaths in Infancy: 5th Annual Report, 1 January–31 December 1996.* London: Maternal and Child Health Research Consortium; 1998.

35. Leung TY, Stuart O, Sahota DS, Suen SS, Lau TK, Lao TT. Head-to-body delivery interval and risk of fetal acidosis and hypoxic ischaemic encephalopathy in shoulder dystocia: a retrospective review. *BJOG* 2011; 118: 474–9.

36. Metaizeau JP, Gayet C, Plenat F. [Brachial plexus birth injuries. An experimental study (author's transl)]. *Chir Pediatr* 1979; 20: 159–63. Article in French.

37. MacKenzie IZ, Shah M, Lean K, Dutton S, Newdick H, Tucker DE. Management of shoulder dystocia: trends in incidence and maternal and neonatal morbidity. *Obstet Gynecol* 2007; 110: 1059–68.

38. Crofts J, Lenguerrand E, Bentham G, Tawfik S, Claireaux H, Odd D. Prevention of brachial plexus injury – 12 years of shoulder dystocia training: an interrupted time-series study. *JOG* 2015; Feb 17. doi: 10.1111/1471-0528.13302.

Module 10
Umbilical cord prolapse

Key learning points

■ Recognize the risk factors for umbilical cord prolapse.

■ Call for appropriate help.

■ Perform maneuvers to reduce cord compression.

■ Communicate effectively with the patient and the team.

■ Understand the importance of appropriate documentation.

Common difficulties observed in training drills

■ Recognition of occult cord prolapse.

■ Inappropriate handling of the cord.

■ Delay moving the patient to an appropriate position to relieve cord compression.

■ Not calling for appropriate help.

■ Omitting umbilical cord gases after delivery.

Introduction

Umbilical cord prolapse is defined as descent of the cord through the cervix, either alongside (occult) or past (overt) the presenting part, in the presence of ruptured membranes. The incidence of umbilical cord prolapse ranges from 0.1 to 0.6% of all births.[1,2,3] It is increased to around 1% with breech presentations.[4]

Risk factors for cord prolapse

Cord prolapse occurs after rupture of the amniotic membranes (spontaneously or artificially) when the fetal presenting part is poorly applied to the cervix. The umbilical cord slips below the presenting part and may be compressed, compromising the fetal blood supply.

The presence of risk factors (Box 10.1) should raise suspicion, but the occurrence of cord prolapse remains extremely unpredictable. A common feature of all the risk factors is a poorly applied fetal presenting part.

Prevention

It has been suggested in the past that women with transverse, oblique, or unstable lie be offered elective admission to hospital at 37 weeks (or sooner if there are signs of labor or suspicion of ruptured membranes)[5,6] before planned cesarean section at term. Though elective admission would not prevent cord prolapse per se, it would place the patient in a location for immediate diagnosis and treatment if prolapse occurs, improving neonatal outcome. This practice clearly would not be cost effective and has not become common.

Artificial rupture of membranes should be avoided if the cord is palpable on vaginal examination (funic presentation).[5] Any obstetric intervention after membrane rupture (e.g., application of fetal scalp electrode, manual rotation of vertex, internal podalic version) carries a risk of cord prolapse, and upward displacement of the presenting part should be minimized after rupture.

Box 10.1 Risk factors for cord prolapse

Antenatal	Intrapartum
Breech presentation	Amniotomy (especially with a high presenting part)
Unstable lie	Prematurity
Oblique or transverse lie	Breech presentation
Polyhydramnios	Internal podalic version
External cephalic version	Second twin
Expectant management of premature rupture of membranes	Elevation of the fetal head during a rotational assisted delivery
Previous cord prolapse	Fetal scalp electrode application

Artificial rupture of the membranes should be avoided when the presenting part is unengaged and/or mobile. If artificial rupture is necessary, combined fundal and suprapubic pressure and/or stabilization of a longitudinal lie may reduce the risk of cord prolapse. It is advantageous to rupture the membranes in or near the operating room where there are facilities to perform an immediate emergency cesarean section if required.

Perinatal complications

The maternal mortality rate associated with umbilical cord prolapse has fallen over the last century, but remains high (approximately 9%).[2] Cases of cord prolapse are still consistently featured in perinatal mortality reviews.

The interval between diagnosis and birth is significantly related to stillbirth and perinatal death. Cord prolapse outside hospital carries a worse prognosis, and the delay associated with transfer to the hospital is a contributory factor should cord prolapse complicate a home or free standing birthing center delivery.[2,7,8,9] Women should be informed of these potential complications when choosing to have their baby outside the hospital.

Infants may experience birth asphyxia due to umbilical cord compression and/or arterial vasospasm secondary to the exposure to vaginal fluids and/or air, resulting in hypoxic–ischemic encephalopathy, cerebral palsy, or neonatal death.[10] However, perinatal death after umbilical cord prolapse is more commonly related to the complications of prematurity than intrapartum asphyxia.[2,11]

Management of umbilical cord prolapse

An outline for the management of cord prolapse is shown in Figure 10.1. This is described in detail in the next section.

Recognize – cord prolapse

Early diagnosis is important. Cord prolapse may be obvious when there is a loop of umbilical cord protruding through the vulva. However, cord prolapse is not always apparent and may only be detected on vaginal examination.

Cord prolapse should be suspected when there is an abnormal fetal heart rate pattern (e.g., bradycardia, decelerations) in the presence of ruptured membranes, particularly if they begin soon after membrane rupture. A speculum and/or a digital vaginal examination should be performed when cord prolapse is suspected, regardless of gestation. Mismanagement of

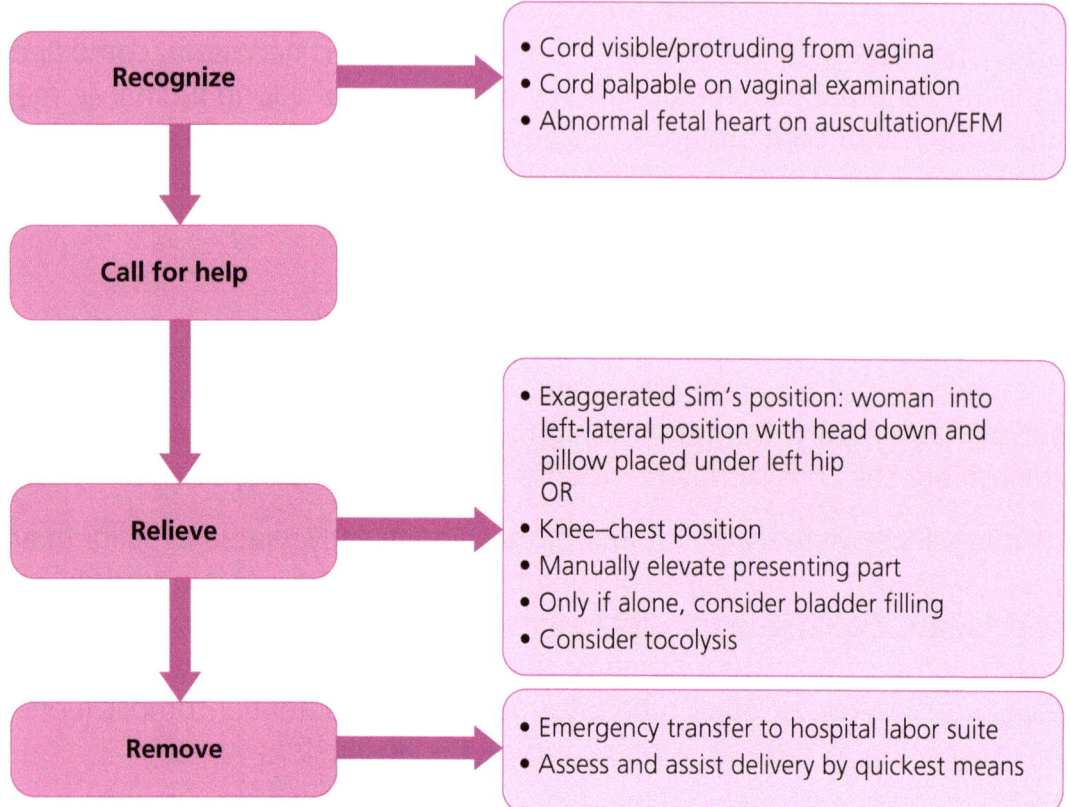

Figure 10.1 Outline of management of cord prolapse

abnormal fetal heart rate patterns is one of the most common aspects of substandard care identified in perinatal death associated with cord prolapse.[5]

Call for help

Call for help as soon as a cord prolapse is diagnosed, including (if possible) a senior labor nurse or midwife, additional staff, the most experienced obstetrician available, an anesthesiologist, the operating room team, and the neonatal team.

Should cord prolapse occur outside of the hospital, an ambulance should be called immediately to transfer the woman to the nearest obstetric unit. Even if delivery appears imminent, an ambulance should still be called to help with any neonatal compromise.

When help arrives, "cord prolapse" should be stated clearly so all in attendance immediately understand the problem. Caregivers outside the obstetric unit (nurses, ambulance staff, general practitioners) should speak directly with the obstetric unit, clearly stating that they are transferring a woman with a cord prolapse and provide an estimated time of arrival. This will ensure the appropriate hospital-based providers are aware and prepared for a timely delivery on arrival.

Relieve – cord compression

Elevate the presenting part as soon as a cord prolapse is recognized to minimize compression. This is best done by digital elevation of the presenting part but, if there is no help, may be assisted by maternal positioning and bladder filling. Tocolysis may also be useful if uterine activity is present.

Maternal positioning

The knee–chest face-down position is traditionally recommended for the management of umbilical cord prolapse. However, this position is less suitable for transportation and the exaggerated Sim's position (left-lateral with a pillow under the left hip) with or without Trendelenburg (bed tilted so that the woman's head is lower than the pelvis) is an alternative (Figure 10.2).

Manual elevation of the presenting part

If cord prolapse is recognized at the time of membrane rupture, the examiner's fingers should be kept in the vagina to elevate the presenting part, thus reducing compression of the cord, particularly during contractions. If the umbilical cord has prolapsed out of the vagina, attempt to gently replace it back into the vagina with minimal handling. There is no evidence to support the practice of covering the exposed cord with sterile gauze soaked in warmed saline.

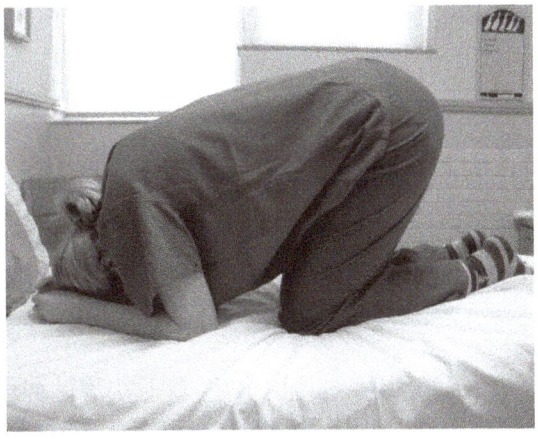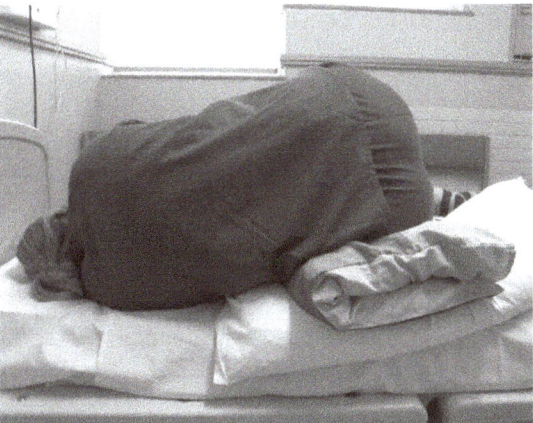

Figure 10.2 Maternal positioning to aid elevation of presenting part: (a) knee–chest; (b) exaggerated Sim's position

Reduce contractions

Stop any oxytocin infusion immediately. Tocolysis (terbutaline 250 mcg sc) has been used to reduce contractions and improve fetal bradycardia when there is a cord prolapse.[5,12,13]

Bladder filling

Bladder filling was first proposed by Vago in 1970[14] as a method of relieving pressure on the umbilical cord. In theory, bladder filling raises the presenting part of the fetus off the compressed cord for an extended period of time, thereby eliminating the need for an examiner's fingers to displace the presenting part.[15] Existing studies are conflicting.

If the decision-to-birth interval is likely to be prolonged, particularly if it involves ambulance transfer into hospital, elevation of the presenting part by bladder filling may be considered. A Foley catheter is placed into the bladder. The bladder is then filled via the catheter with sterile (0.9%) saline using an intravenous blood infusion set. The catheter should be clamped after 500 to 750 ml has been instilled. It is essential to empty the bladder just before any method of delivery is attempted.

> **Any of the measures described above may be useful during preparation for delivery; however, birth should not be delayed by trying to implement these measures.**

Assessment of fetal wellbeing

Continuous electronic fetal monitoring should be performed. An ultrasound scan should be performed if there is no audible fetal heart beat before cesarean delivery.

Remove – transport and assist birth

Cord prolapse should be managed in a unit with full anesthetic and neonatal services. Immediate transfer is essential if cord prolapse occurs outside a labor suite.

Good communication is required so that appropriate healthcare providers are ready to receive the mother on transfer and the operating room is on standby. If there is no intravenous access, place a large-bore intravenous cannula (14/16-gauge) and take blood for a type and hold plus a CBC.

Assessment for birth

- If the cervix is not fully dilated, cesarean section should be performed.

- If the cervix is fully dilated, consider an assisted vaginal birth as long as it is anticipated delivery can be accomplished quickly and safely. Vacuum or forceps should be considered only if the prerequisites for operative vaginal delivery are otherwise met.

- Breech extraction may be performed under some circumstances, for example after internal podalic version for the second twin.

In general, poor perinatal outcomes are associated with difficult attempts at achieving vaginal delivery. The impact of delay could be exacerbated by the possible need to perform a cesarean after a failed instrumental delivery.

The use of temporary measures to relieve pressure on the cord, as described in the previous section, should enable an attempt at regional anesthesia (spinal or epidural top-up). However, prolonged and repeated attempts at regional anesthesia must be avoided. The presenting part should be kept elevated while anesthesia is undertaken. Clear communication about the urgency and timing of birth is required between the nursing, obstetric, and anesthetic teams to ensure the safest method of anesthesia is used for both mother and fetus.

Neonatal resuscitation

An experienced neonatal team must be present at birth to ensure full cardiorespiratory support is available for the neonate, if required. Paired umbilical cord gases should be taken after birth to document the neonatal condition.

Documentation

The medical record should include the time the cord prolapse either occurred or was discovered, the time help was called and arrived, the methods used to alleviate cord compression, the time of the decision to assist the delivery and method, and the time of birth. A template that may aid documentation is provided in Figure 10.3.

Parents

Cord prolapse is a frightening experience for the parents. It is important to explain what is happening and to give the mother clear instructions. The parents will need support and debriefing. Clinicians should be encouraged to

PROMPT

PRactical Obstetric Multi-Professional Training

Name.....................................
Date of Birth.........................
Hospital No...........................

Cord Prolapse Documentation template

Please tick the relevant boxes

Labor floor superviser called: Yes   ☐   No   ☐

Time called:.....................   Time arrived:.......................   Name:..............................

Obstetrician called: Yes   ☐   No   ☐

Time called:.....................   Time arrived:.......................   Name:..............................

Neonatologist called: Yes   ☐   No   ☐

Time called:...................   Time arrived:.......................   Name:..............................

Diagnosed at home or hospital: Home ☐   Hospital ☐

Time of diagnosis:...........................

Cervical dilatation at diagnosis:........... cm

Procedures used in managing cord prolapse				
Elevating the presenting part manually	Yes ☐		No ☐	
Left lateral, head tilt down / Knee-Chest position	(Please circle)			
Tocolysis with sc Terbutaline	Yes ☐		No ☐	
Filling the bladder	Yes ☐		No ☐	

Mode of birth		Mode of Anesthesia	
Normal	☐	GA	☐
Forceps	☐	Spinal	☐
Vacuum	☐	Epidural	☐
C/S	☐		
Other	☐		

Diagnosis to birth interval:...........................minutes

Neonatal outcome		
Apgar Scores:	**Weight:**....................kg	
1 min:	**Cord pH**	**Base Excess**
5 mins:	Venous:	
10 mins:	Arterial:	

Admission to NICU:
Yes ☐   No ☐   Reason:...

Known Risk Factors? Please state:...

	Follow–up appointment offered?
Mother debriefed Yes ☐ No ☐	

Signature:.....................................   Print:...

Designation:...............................   Date:...

Figure 10.3 Example of cord prolapse documentation template

visit the parents the following day and subsequently, if required, to discuss events, answer any questions, and address concerns.

Training

With regular training, the maneuvers to relieve cord compression can be conducted efficiently without delaying birth. A retrospective study examined the effect of team rehearsals, and the introduction of regular training was associated with both more frequent actions to relieve cord compression and a shorter diagnosis-to-birth interval; crucially, it was also associated with consistently better neonatal outcomes.[16]

Key points

- Cord prolapse is a life-threatening complication for the perinate.
- Once a cord prolapse is recognized:
  - relieve the pressure on the cord
  - move the mother to an appropriate place for delivery
  - deliver the baby by the safest and most expedient means.
- Document your actions clearly and legibly.
- Discuss events with the parents.

References

1. Critchlow CW, Leet TL, Benedetti TJ, Daling JR. Risk factors and infant outcomes associated with umbilical cord prolapse: a population-based case-control study among births in Washington State. *Am J Obstet Gynecol* 1994; 170: 613–18.

2. Gibbons C, O'Herlihy C, Murphy CF. Umbilical cord prolapse – changing patterns and improved outcomes: a retrospective cohort study. *Br J Obstet Gynecol* 2014; 121: 1705–8.

3. Lin MG. Umbilical cord prolapse. *Obstetrical & Gynecological Survey* 2006; 61: 269–77.

4. Panter KR, Hannah ME. Umbilical cord prolapse: so far so good? *Lancet* 1996; 347: 74.

5. Royal College of Obstetricians and Gynaecologists. *Umbilical Cord Prolapse*. Green-top Guideline No. 50. London: RCOG; 2014.

6. Phelan JP, Boucher M, Mueller E, McCart D, Horenstein J, Clark S. The nonlaboring transverse lie. A management dilemma. *J Reprod Med* 1986; 31: 184–6.

7. Beard RJ, Johnson DA. Fetal distress due to cord prolapse through a fenestration in a lower segment uterine scar. *J Obstet Gynaecol Br Commonw* 1972; 79: 763.

8. Johnson KC, Daviss BA. Outcomes of planned home births with certified professional midwives: large prospective study in North America. *BMJ* 2005; 330: 1416.

9. *Breech Presentation at Onset of Labour. Confidential Enquiries into Stillbirths and Deaths in Infancy. 7th Annual Report*. London: Maternal and Child Health Consortium; 2000.

10. MacLennan A. A template for defining a causal relation between acute intrapartum events and cerebral palsy: international consensus statement. *BMJ* 1999; 319: 1054–9.

11. Ylä-Outinen A, Heinonen PK, Tuimala R. Predisposing and risk factors of umbilical cord prolapse. *Acta Obstet Gynecol Scand* 1985; 64: 567–70.

12. Gruese ME, Prickett SA. Nursing management of umbilical cord prolaspe. *J Obstet Gynecol Neonatal Nurs* 1993; 22: 311–15.

13. Katz Z, Shoham Z, Lancet M, Blickstein I, Mogilner BM, Zalel Y. Management of labor with umbilical cord prolapse: a 5-year study. *Obstet Gynecol* 1988; 72: 278–81.

14. Vago T. Prolapse of the umbilical cord: a method of management. *Am J Obstet Gynecol* 1970; 107: 967–9.

15. Caspi E, Lotan Y, Schreyer P. Prolapse of the cord: reduction of perinatal mortality by bladder instillation and cesarean section. *Isr J Med Sci* 1983; 19: 541–5.

16. Siassakos D, Hasafa Z, Sibanda T, Fox R, Donald F, Winter C, et al. Retrospective cohort study of diagnosis–delivery interval with umbilical cord prolapse: the effect of team training. *BJOG* 2009; 116: 1089–96.

Module 11
Vaginal breech birth

Key learning points

- Ensure continuous electronic fetal monitoring (EFM) in labor (which is continued after any decision to perform a cesarean delivery).
- Ensure full cervical dilation before pushing.
- Await visualization of the breech at the perineum before encouraging active pushing.
- Take a **"hands off"** approach as much as possible – allow the breech to "deliver itself."
- Avoid traction on the breech.
- Understand the maneuvers that may be required to assist a breech birth.

Common difficulties observed in training drills

- Active intervention.
- Premature initiation of assisted breech maneuvers.
- Pressure on non-bony prominences during those maneuvers.

Introduction

The incidence of breech presentation at term is 3 to 4%, although it is much higher earlier in pregnancy (at 28 weeks, 20% of fetuses are breech presentation). Breech presentation is associated with a higher perinatal morbidity and mortality than cephalic presentation regardless of the delivery route: prematurity, congenital malformations, birth asphyxia, and trauma are all more common with breech presentations.[1] Such risk factors guide antenatal, intrapartum, and neonatal management.

Definition

Breech presentation is one where the presenting part of the fetus is either the buttocks or lower limb(s); the breech can be extended, flexed, or footling (Figure 11.1).

(a)

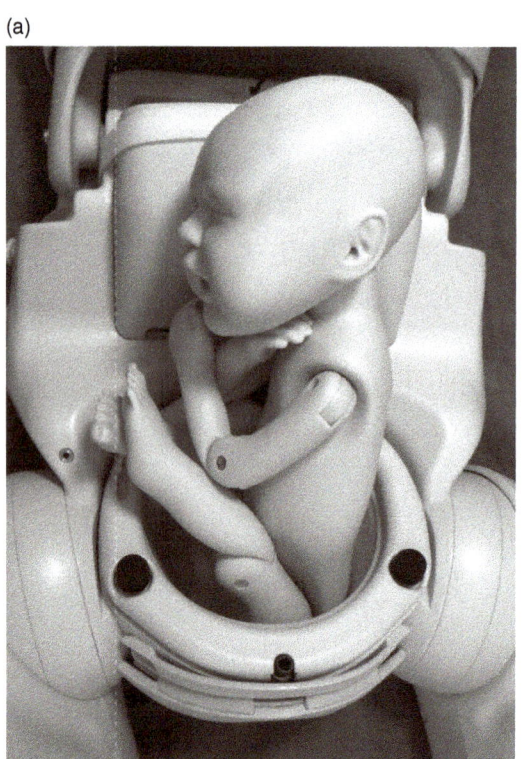

(b)

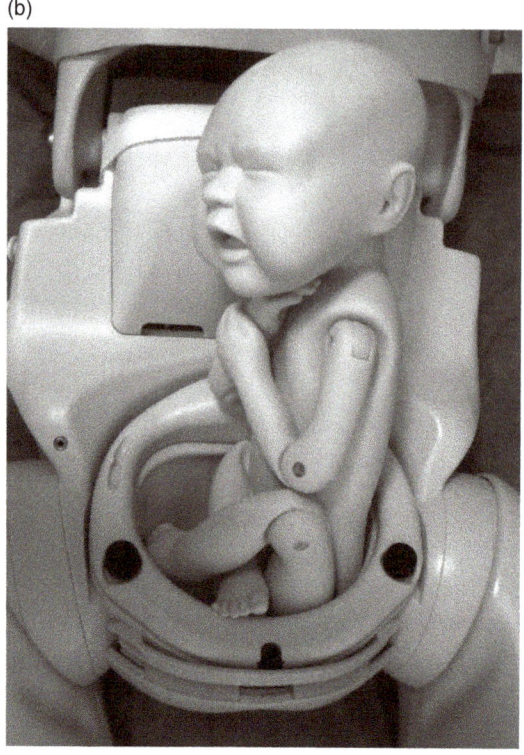

(c)

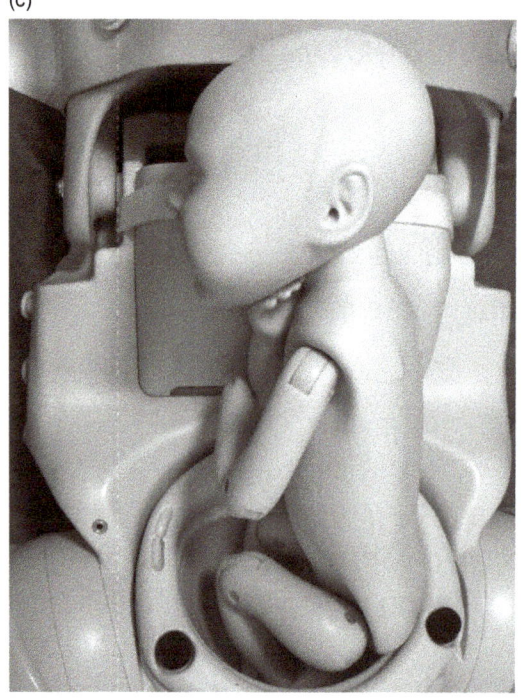

Figure 11.1 Types of breech presentation and incidence: (a) frank (65%): hips flexed, knees extended; (b) complete (10%): hips flexed, knees flexed, and feet not below the buttocks; (c) footling (25%): feet or knees are lowest (either single or double footling)

Predisposing factors

Factors that predispose to a breech presentation are listed in Box 11.1.

The rate of vaginal breech delivery declined from 1.2% in 1980 to 0.3% in 2001, and has continued to decline as a result of the Term Breech Trial.[2,3,4] This study compared outcomes after planned vaginal and planned cesarean births for breech presentation. It concluded that there was a significant reduction in perinatal morbidity and mortality in the planned cesarean group (reduction in mortality of 75%). In addition, there was no significant increase in maternal morbidity or mortality with planned cesarean births.

This is not to suggest the trial was perfect. The vaginal delivery group ended up with an excess of fetuses with serious/lethal anomalies. Their elimination from analyses would have removed the significant differences that halted the trial. Further, two-year follow-up data from the trial did not demonstrate any significant differences in neurodevelopment between the two groups. As a result, the benefits of routine cesarean delivery remain gray, and it is unclear whether the long-term benefits for the child of a planned cesarean section for breech presentation outweigh the neonatal risks of delivery without labor, and the maternal risks of subsequent additional cesareans.

Despite the increasing practice of obstetricians to deliver breech fetuses by cesarean, it is essential that practitioners develop, maintain, and practice their skills for assisted vaginal breech births. Firstly, the same maneuvers are employed for breech delivery during cesarean section. Secondly, the optimal mode of birth for women in advanced labor or preterm labor with a breech presentation remains unclear, and vaginal birth is an option and sometimes necessary. And, lastly, there is no advantage to cesarean delivery of the non-vertex second twin between 32 weeks and term.[5] Recommendations for mode of birth are shown in Box 11.2.

Box 11.1 Factors associated with breech presentation

Previous breech delivery	Uterine anomalies
Premature labor	Pelvic tumor or fibroids
High parity	Placenta previa
Multiple pregnancy	Hydrocephaly/anencephaly
Polyhydramnios	Fetal neuromuscular disorders
Oligohydramnios	Fetal head and neck tumors

Box 11.2 Summary of recommendations regarding mode of delivery in breech presentation

- Neonatal morbidity and mortality in the term breech may be reduced by planned cesarean delivery.

- Routine cesarean delivery for the non-vertex second twin does not improve outcome.

- There is no substantative evidence that cesarean delivery of a preterm breech is beneficial.

- There is no evidence that cesarean delivery for a laboring breech is beneficial.

- There is no evidence to support external cephalic version (ECV) for preterm breech.

- There is no evidence of long-term benefit in perinatal outcome for a breech presentation delivered by elective cesarean section.

(Adapted from references 1 and 5)

Management of vaginal breech birth

Types of vaginal breech birth

Spontaneous breech birth:	The fetus is allowed to deliver without assistance or manipulation. This accounts for a small proportion of breech deliveries, most of which are very premature.
Assisted breech birth:	The most common method of vaginal breech birth. The fetus is allowed to descend with the accoucheur employing a "hands off" approach. Recognized maneuvers are used to assist the delivery when required.
Breech extraction:	Mainly reserved for the delivery of the non-vertex second twin. Breech extraction involves grasping one or both of the fetal feet within the uterine cavity and bringing them down through the vagina, before continuing the maneuvers used in an assisted breech birth. Breech extraction should not be attempted in singleton pregnancies, as it is associated with a high rate of birth injury (25%) and mortality (10%).

Management of the first stage of labor

It is recommended that a vaginal breech birth should take place in a hospital with facilities for emergency cesarean section. There is no robust evidence regarding the complications of breech delivery outside the hospital setting.[1]

Preparation

Inform the labor nurse, obstetrician, anesthesiologist, and operating room staff on admission (diagnosis); introduce key staff members to the parents.

Discuss the route of delivery with the patient again and ensure that she still wishes to proceed with a vaginal breech delivery. Discuss analgesia early; the selected method is one more of preference and experience than evidence based.[1] Consider a pudendal block if epidural analgesia is not available. Explain the delivery techniques and that a neonatal team will routinely attend a vaginal breech birth.

Establish intravenous access and obtain blood samples for a CBC and blood type and hold. The labor room and neonatal resuscitation equipment should be immediately available. Ensure that prerequisites for an assisted vaginal breech birth are present, including forceps.

Electronic fetal monitoring

Continuous EFM is recommended for women with a breech presentation during labor and birth. One review of 56 deaths of singleton breech births found clinical evidence of hypoxia before birth in all but one.[2] The report concluded that: "The assessments and decisions made by health professionals, during labor, in particular those regarding intrapartum fetal surveillance, were the critical factors in the avoidable deaths." A fetal scalp electrode can be placed on the fetal buttock if required.[6]

Labor progress

Labor augmentation with oxytocin is considered best avoided, and amniotomy should be performed with caution. A vaginal examination should be performed immediately after spontaneous (or artificial) rupture of the membranes to exclude a cord prolapse.

Management of the second stage of labor

A cesarean section should be undertaken when there is delay in the descent of the breech at any point in the 2nd stage of labor assuming the mother is pushing adequately, as it may be a sign of relative fetopelvic disproportion.[1]

Vaginal breech delivery should take place in the labor suite operating room and be attended by practitioners with adequate experience and skills to assist the birth, if need be. The attendants should include minimally an experience labor nurse, two obstetricians, and a neonatologist. An anesthesiologist and operating room staff should also be present on standby. Allow the breech to "labor down." Active pushing should be encouraged after the breech is visible at the perineum.

> **Remember: allow the breech to spontaneously descend; keep interventions to a minimum.**

Vaginal breech birth: assisted maneuvers

- A vaginal breech delivery ideally requires two people – one accoucheur conducting the actual delivery, and the second helping to guide the fetal head into the pelvis.

- Episiotomy should be used selectively to facilitate birth.[1]

- Spontaneous birth of limbs and trunk is preferable (Figure 11.2a), but the legs may need to be released by applying pressure to the popliteal fossae (Figure 11.2b).

- It is important to ensure that support is provided over the bony prominences of the iliac crests when handling the baby to reduce the risk of soft-tissue/internal injury.

(a)

(b)

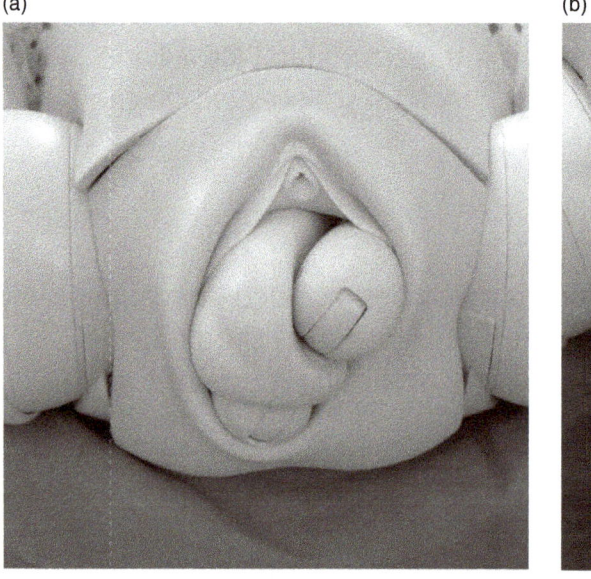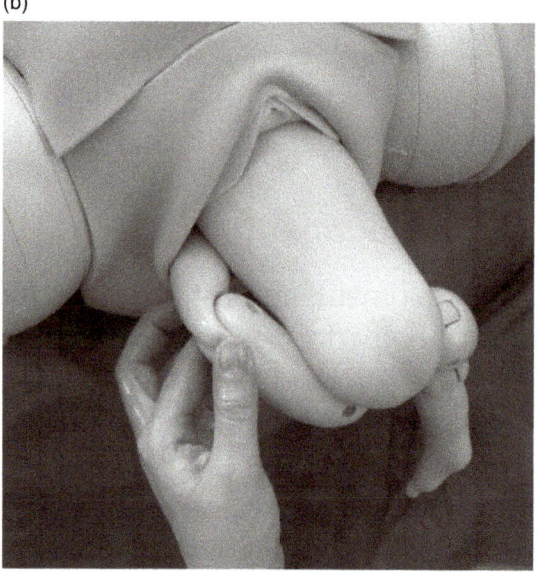

Figure 11.2 (a) Spontaneous birth of the limbs and trunk; (b) applying pressure to the popliteal fossae

- Ensure that the buttocks remain sacrum anterior. Controlled rotation may be required if the trunk appears to be rotating to a sacrum posterior position, but handling of the baby should be only over the bony prominences.
- Avoid handling the umbilical cord as this increases vasospasm.
- Encourage spontaneous birth until the scapulae are visible.
- **Pulling on the infant's trunk can cause a nuchal arm and should be avoided.**
- If the arms are not released spontaneously, use the Løvsett's maneuver, as shown in Figure 11.3.

Engagement in the pelvis of the after-coming head

After releasing the arms, support the baby until the nape of the neck becomes visible, using the weight of the baby to encourage flexion (Figure 11.4). Have your colleague guide the head into the pelvis and then apply suprapubic pressure to assist flexion of the head for delivery.

Mauriceau–Smellie–Veit maneuver

The Mauriceau–Smellie–Veit maneuver may be required to assist delivery of the after-coming head (Figure 11.5). The baby's body should be supported on the flexor surface of the accoucheur's forearm. The first and third finger of the accoucheur's hand should be placed on the cheekbones (though taught in the past, it is probably best to avoid placing the middle finger in the fetal mouth as fetal injury has been reported). With the other hand, apply pressure to the occiput with the middle finger and place the other fingers simultaneously on the fetal shoulders to promote flexion (i.e., keep the chin on the chest) (Figure 11.6).

Burns–Marshall technique

Another way of assisting the birth of the head is to raise the body vertically and have an assistant hold the baby's feet (Burns–Marshall technique). Sometimes, this will promote spontaneous birth of the head (Figure 11.7). Concern has been voiced about the risks of the Burns–Marshall method if used incorrectly, as it may lead to overextension of the baby's neck.[1]

Forceps to assist birth of the head

Delivery of the fetal head can be assisted with forceps. An assistant should hold the baby level while the forceps are applied from underneath the fetal

(a)
(b)
(c)
(d)

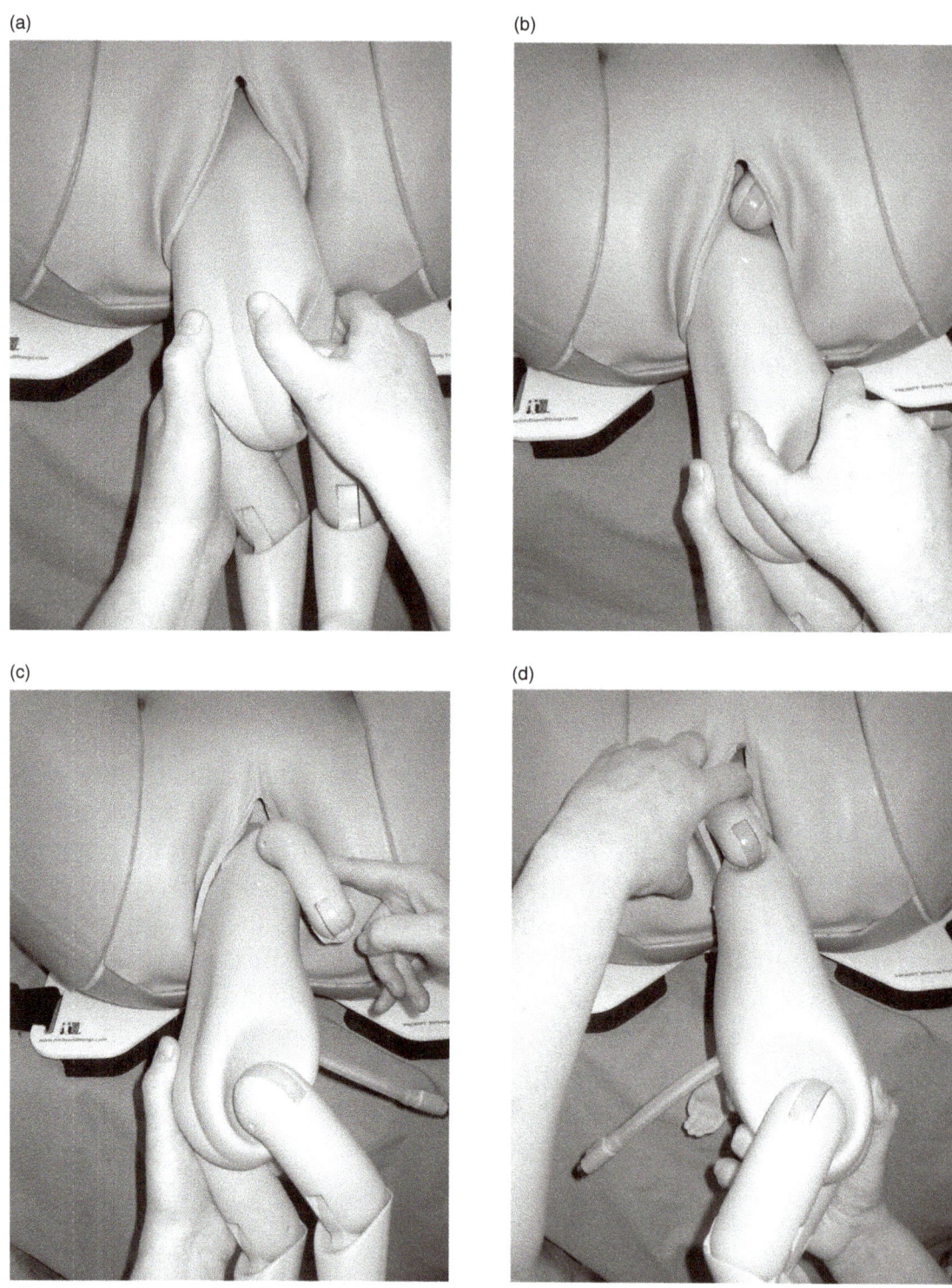

Figure 11.3 Løvsett's maneuver. (a) Gently hold the baby over the bony prominences of the hips and sacrum and rotate the baby so that one arm is uppermost (anterior). (b and c) Release the upper arm by placing an index finger over the baby's shoulder and follow the infant's arm to the antecubital fossa. The arm is then flexed for delivery. (d) Following release of the first arm, rotate the baby 180 degrees, keeping the back uppermost, so that the second arm is now upper. Release this arm as described in (b).

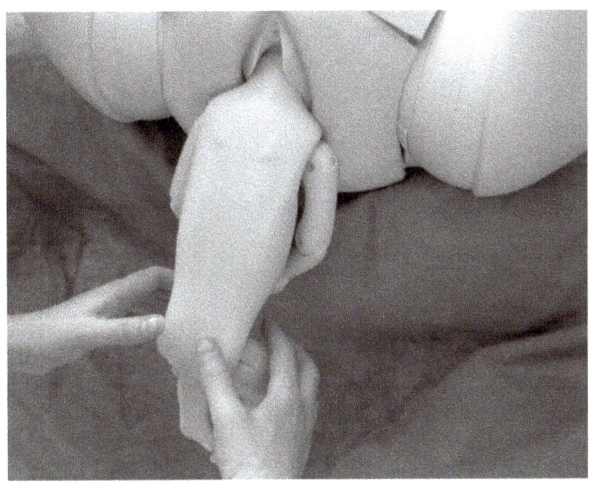

Figure 11.4 Nape of neck visible: using the weight of the baby to encourage flexion

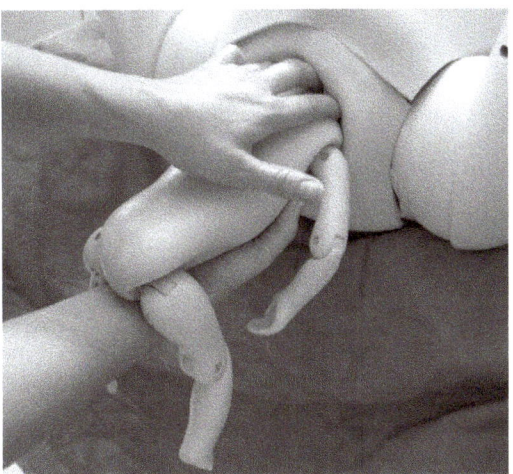

Figure 11.5 The Mauriceau–Smellie–Veit maneuver for delivery of the after-coming head

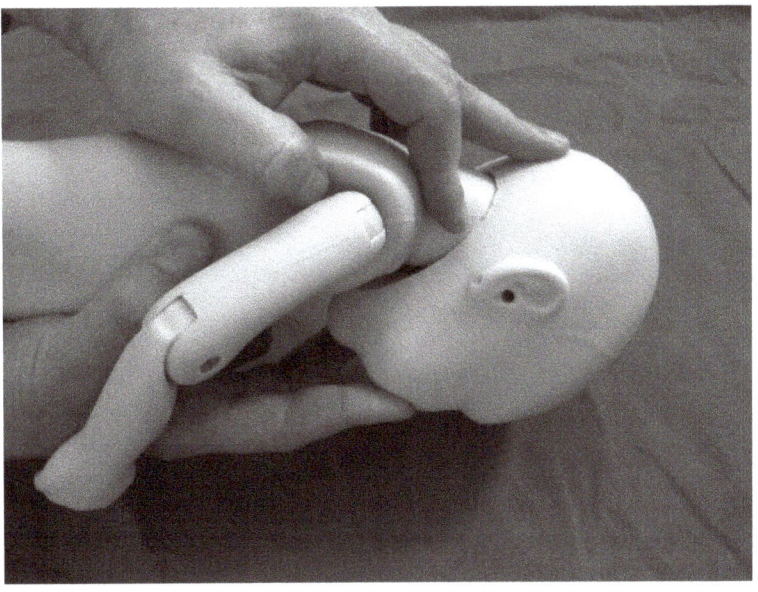

Figure 11.6 Flexion and birth of the fetal head using the Mauriceau–Smellie–Veit maneuver

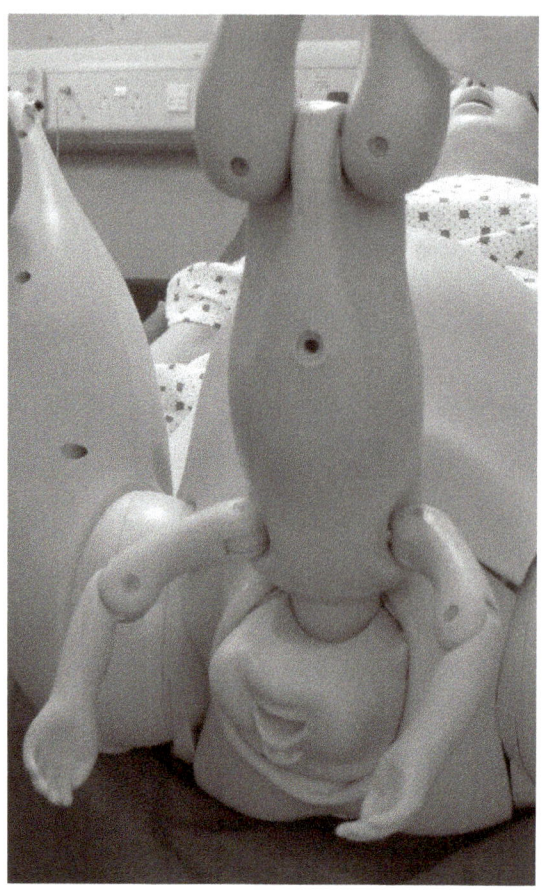

Figure 11.7 The Burns–Marshall technique for delivering the head

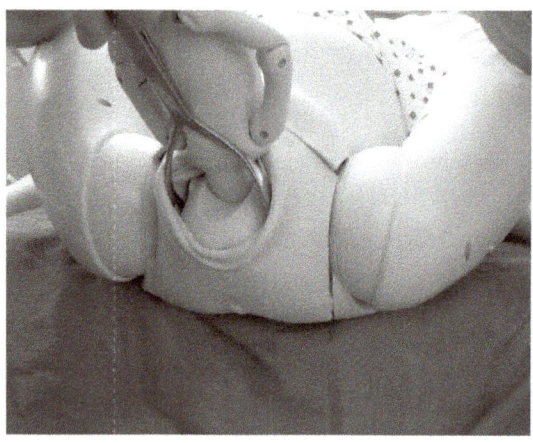 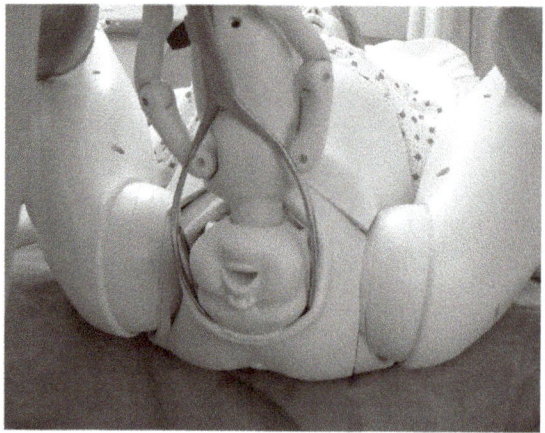

Figure 11.8 Kielland forceps to assist birth of the head

body. The axis of traction should aim to flex the head (Figure 11.8). There is debate over which type of forceps is best; Kielland, Rhodes', Piper's, and Wrigley's forceps have all been reported. There is no experimental evidence to indicate one is preferable over another, and previous experience of the practitioner is likely to be the most important factor.

Complications and potential solutions

Failure to assist birth of the after-coming head

If conservative methods and forceps fail to assist birth of the head, successful births have been reported with symphysiotomy or rapid cesarean section.[1]

Head entrapment during a preterm breech delivery

The major cause of head entrapment is the passage of the preterm fetal trunk through an incompletely dilated cervix. In this situation, the cervix can be incised to release the head. The incisions are made at the 10 and 2 o'clock positions to avoid the cervical neurovascular bundles that run laterally in the cervix. Care should be taken as extension into the lower segment of the uterus can occur.[7]

Nuchal arms

This is when one or both of arms become extended and trapped behind the fetal head. Nuchal arms complicate up to 5% of breech births (Figure 11.9) and may be caused by early traction on the breech. There is significant morbidity associated with nuchal arms (e.g., brachial plexus injuries); early traction on the breech should be avoided.

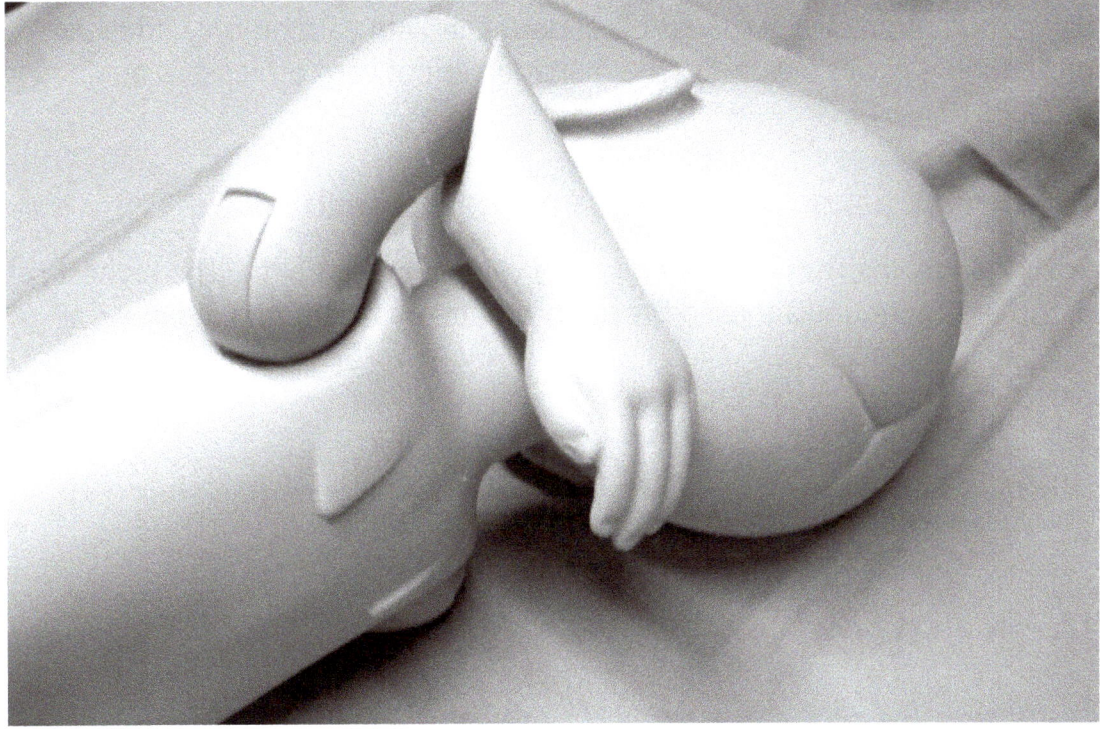

Figure 11.9 Nuchal arm

> ### Box 11.3 Fetal risks associated with vaginal breech birth
>
> Intrapartum death
>
> Intracranial hemorrhage
>
> Hypoxic ischemic encephalopathy
>
> Brachial plexus injury
>
> Rupture of the liver, kidney, or spleen
>
> Dislocation of the neck, shoulder, or hip
>
> Fractured clavicle, humerus, or femur
>
> Cord prolapse
>
> Occipital diastasis and cerebellar injury

Nuchal arms are released using Løvsett's maneuver. Here the accoucheur runs their finger along the fetal arm to the antecubital fossa, applies pressure to flex and release the arm for delivery.

Cord prolapse

Cord prolapse is more common with all breech presentations, especially the footling breech (10–25%). The most important factor with cord prolapse is prevention. Amniotomy should be undertaken with caution only after the presenting part fills the pelvis. The management of cord prolapse is outlined in Module 10.

Fetal risks associated with vaginal breech birth

Box 11.3 lists the risks associated with a vaginal breech birth. The highest risk group are those undiagnosed breech presentations identified in labor.[2]

Further reading

James DK, Steer PJ, Weiner CP, Gonik B. *High Risk Pregnancy: Management Options*, 4th edn. London: Saunders; 2011.

References

1. Royal College of Obstetricians and Gynaecologists. *The Management of Breech Presentation*. Green-top Guideline No. 20b. London: RCOG; 2006 [www.rcog.org.uk/womens-health/clinical-guidance/management-breech-presentation-green-top-20b].

2. Maternal and Child Health Research Consortium. *Confidential Enquiry into Stillbirths and Deaths in Infancy: 7th Annual Report, 1 January–31 December 1998*. London: Maternal and Child Health Research Consortium; 2000.

3. Department of Health. *NHS Maternity Statistics, England: 2001–02*. Bulletin 2003/09, 2002 [www.dh.gov.uk/en/Publicationsandstatistics/Statistics/StatisticalWorkAreas/Statisticalhealthcar e/DH_4086520].

4. Hannah ME, Hannah WJ, Hewson SA, Hodnett ED, Saigal S, Willan AR. Planned caesarean section versus planned vaginal birth for breech presentation at term: a randomised multicentre trial. Term Breech Trial Collaborative Group. *Lancet* 2002; 356: 1375–83.

5. Barrett JF, Hannah ME, Hutton EK, Willan AR, Allen AC, Armson BA, et al. A randomized trial of planned cesarean or vaginal delivery for twin pregnancy. *N Engl J Med* 2013; 369(14): 1295–305.

6. National Collaborating Centre for Women's and Children's Health. *Intrapartum Care: Care of Healthy Women and their Babies during Childbirth*. Clinical Guideline. London: RCOG Press; 2007.

7. Robertson PA, Foran CM, Croughan-Minihane MS, Kilpatrick SJ. Head entrapment and neonatal outcome by mode of delivery in breech deliveries from 28 to 36 weeks of gestation. *Am J Obstet Gynecol* 1996; 174: 1742–7.

Module 12
Twin birth

Common difficulties observed in training drills

- Failing to prepare the room for delivery in advance.
- If spontaneous delivery of the second twin is planned, failure to maintain a longitudinal lie of the second twin until the presenting part has engaged into the pelvis.
- Premature amniotomy if spontaneous delivery of the second twin is planned.

Introduction

"Non-identical" (dizygotic) twins are the most common type of twinning and result from fertilization of two eggs (ova). Dizygotic twins are genetically no more similar than siblings, having separate placental circulations and gestational sacs (dizygotic, diamniotic, dichorionic).

"Identical" (monozygotic) twins are less common. They result from the splitting of a single developing embryo and are essentially genetically identical. The degree of separation depends on the developmental stage at which the split takes place, and can be anything from completely separate circulations (monozygotic, dichorionic, diamniotic) to conjoined twins (monozygotic, monochorionic, monoamniotic).[1] Around one-third of twin pregnancies have a monochorionic placenta.

The incidence of monozygotic twins is fairly constant worldwide. The rate of dizygotic twins varies considerably and there has been an increase due to both the use of fertility treatments and the rising number of older mothers.[2]

All twins share increased risks of preterm birth and fetal growth restriction. Because 100% of monochorionic diamniotic twins have abnormal vessel connections that join the twins' circulations, they have additional risks of twin-to-twin transfusion syndrome, twin anemia polycythemia syndrome (TAPS), and unequal placental sharing.

The perinatal mortality rate of twins is seven times that of singletons and almost every obstetric complication is more common. Much of the excess perinatal mortality is attributable to antepartum events, though some is related to problems during labor and at birth. Box 12.1 lists some of the risks of twin pregnancies both antenatally and in labor.

Box 12.1 Risks of twin pregnancies

Fetal growth restriction

Preterm labor (50% of twins deliver preterm)

Twin-to-twin transfusion (in monochorionic pregnancies)

Malpresentation

Cord prolapse

Cord entanglement (monochorionic, monoamniotic)

Neonatal seizures

Increased respiratory morbidity

Increased risk of cerebral palsy (four times the risk of a singleton pregnancy)

Postpartum hemorrhage for mother

The patient and her partner should be counseled regarding the mode and management of their twin delivery prior to the onset of labor.

Presentation

Approximately 30% of twins present as cephalic/cephalic[3] (Figure 12.1), 35% of twins present as cephalic/non-cepahlic[4] (Figure 12.2), and the remaining 25% of twins present with the leading baby in a non-cephalic presentation at birth[4] (Figures 12.3 and 12.4).

Mode of birth

The optimal route of delivery for twin pregnancies has grown clearer over the past decade – there is no advantage to routine cesarean delivery. The Twin Birth Study compared vaginal to cesarean delivery from 32 to 38 weeks on an intention-to-treat basis. When the first twin was vertex and the second non-cephalic,[4] there were no differences in the rates of adverse perinatal outcome for the second twin whether delivered vaginally or by cesarean section.

The route of delivery is influenced by presentation, amnionicity and chorionicity, predicted fetal weight, gestation, and fetal and maternal wellbeing.[1] A vaginal delivery should be offered in otherwise uncomplicated twin pregnancies when the first twin is vertex, assuming there are no other relative or absolute contraindications to vaginal birth. It is important to emphasize to the mother that serious, acute intrapartum problems following the birth of the first twin (for example conversion to transverse lie, cord prolapse, prolonged time interval to birth of the second twin) may lead to emergency cesarean delivery. Perinatal death and neonatal morbidity can occur even in cephalic/cephalic presentations.

Most obstetricians will offer an elective cesarean delivery when the first twin is not vertex. This recommendation was abstractly reinforced by the findings of the Term Breech Trial (singletons only), which concluded there was increased morbidity and mortality with vaginal breech birth in singleton pregnancies (see Module 11).[5] It is also widely accepted that monoamniotic and conjoined twins should be delivered by elective cesarean section.[6]

Timing of birth

The majority of women with a twin pregnancy enter spontaneously labor by 37 weeks. There is no robust evidence to base the optimal timing of birth of either identical/monochorionic or non-identical/dichorionic twin pregnancies, but the incidence of stillbirth in twins does rise after 37 to 38 weeks and exceeds that

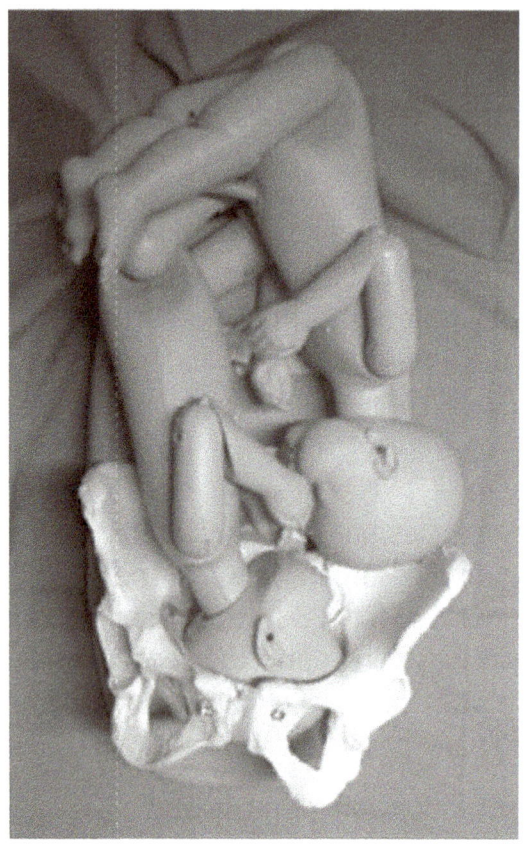

Figure 12.1 Cephalic/cephalic

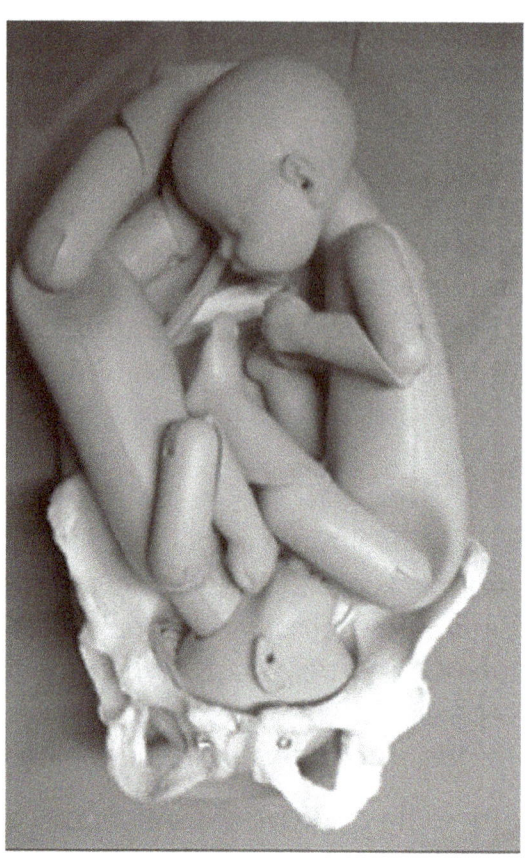

Figure 12.2 Cephalic/breech

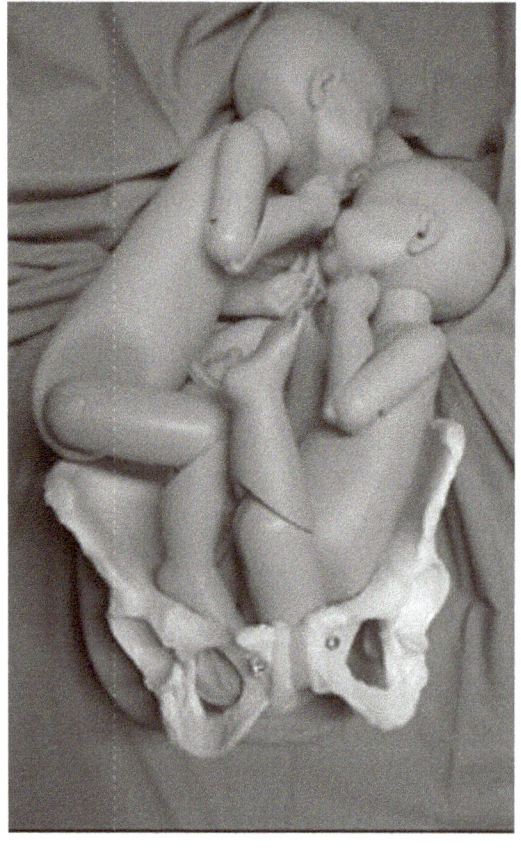

Figure 12.3 Breech/breech

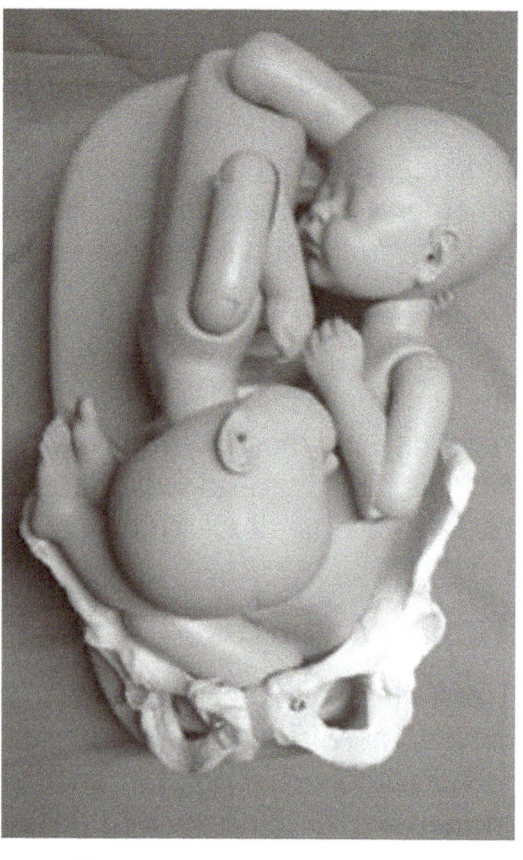

Figure 12.4 Breech/cephalic

of singleton pregnancies.[7] For that reason, delivery should be planned at 37 to 38 weeks of gestation in otherwise uncomplicated dichorionic twin pregnancies and at 36 to 37 weeks of gestation in otherwise uncomplicated monochorionic twin pregnancies.[8]

Management of vaginal twin birth

All women should discuss in the antenatal period with their obstetrician the planned intrapartum care. These discussions should be documented in the medical record.

The discussion should include:

- the increased risk of morbidity for the second twin regardless of the route of delivery
- analgesia, including the advantages and disadvantages of epidural anesthesia
- stabilization of the fetal lie if a spontaneous delivery of the second twin is planned
- the use of oxytocin to augment contractions during the inter-twin period if a spontaneous delivery of twin B is planned
- the possibility of intervention to expedite birth of the second twin (e.g., breech extraction with or without internal podalic version)
- the small risk of cesarean section even after the successful vaginal birth of the first twin
- active management of the 3rd stage of labor and the use of an oxytocin infusion to reduce the risk of postpartum hemorrhage.

First stage of labor

All laboring women with a multiple pregnancy should have one-on-one nursing and be cared for by an experienced obstetrician. The anesthesiologist, neonatologist, and neonatal care unit should be informed of the mother's admission. A clear plan should be documented in the notes. An example of an admission checklist is given in Figure 12.5.

Fetal scalp blood sampling of twin A may be performed if indicated. But if there are concerns for the wellbeing of twin B, then a cesarean section is indicated.

Oxytocin augmentation is not contraindicated for hypotonic contractions in labor.

	Tick when completed	Comments
Introduce the parents to the team.		
Review the prenatal notes including the care plan to identify any antenatal risk factors.		
Explain the plan for delivery.		
Establish intravenous access, take blood for CBC and type and hold.		
Confirm presentation of both twins with ultrasound.		
Continuous electronic fetal monitoring is recommended: • A scalp electrode may be used for twin A to help differentiate the fetal heart recordings. • Ultrasound can be used to identify the optimal location placement of the EFM transducers. • A suitable monitor should be used to enable the differentiation of the two fetal heart tracings.		
Discuss analgesia. An epidural will facilitate any intrauterine manipulation of twin B and can be used for cesarean section if needed.		
Consider giving ranitidine 150 mg PO every 6 hours.		
Obstetrician to document a care plan for twin delivery		
Date:　　　　　　Name:　　　　　　　　　Signature:		

Figure 12.5 An example of a checklist on admission to labor floor

Second stage of labor

The delivery of twins is best performed, or at least supervised, by an experienced obstetrician. Healthcare professionals attending the birth should include:

- at least two labor nurses (preferably experienced)
- at least one additional obstetrician
- at least two members of the neonatal team
- an anesthesiologist.

Box 12.2 Equipment required for a twin delivery

Ultrasound scanner

Lithotomy set (if in OR)

Cesarean delivery pack

Forceps and vacuum

Twin pack (two sets of cord clamps)

Four cord blood-sampling syringes

Two infant warmers with two sets of baby linen and hats

Oxytocin for augmentation after the first twin if a spontaneous delivery of twin B is planned

Oxytocin (40 units in 500 ml normal saline for prophylactic use after 3rd stage of labor) and or methylergonovine for 3rd stage of labor as appropriate

Prepare the delivery room and required healthcare staff in advance so there is a calm and unhurried approach to the birth.

Prepare the room and staff

Ensure prerequisites for twin delivery are present. A checklist may be helpful. A list of the equipment required is shown in Box 12.2.

An oxytocin infusion should be prepared and initiated after the delivery of twin A if spontaneous delivery of twin B is planned as uterine contractions sometimes decrease or come to a stop at this stage.

Prepare the mother

Keep the mother informed. Explain who will be present at the delivery and also their roles.

Twin delivery – procedure

Delivery of the first twin if cephalic is conducted as in a singleton delivery. There are three possible modes of delivery for twin B: breech extraction including internal podalic version if indicated, a spontaneous vaginal delivery, or an emergency cesarean delivery.

If a breech extraction is planned, it should be initiated immediately after the delivery of the first twin. The key person is the second skilled individual who guides the flexed fetal head into the pelvis and assists with the delivery from above.

If a spontaneous delivery of twin B is planned

After delivery of the first twin, an assistant (preferably an experienced obstetrician) stabilizes the lie of the second twin until the presenting part descends into the pelvis. Here the assistant places both hands on the mother's abdomen and holds the fetus in a longitudinal axis. The presentation of twin B is typically unstable, and the optimal place to monitor its heart rate may be facilitated by an ultrasound scan. There should be continuous EFM of twin B after the delivery of the first twin.

The uterine contractions oftern stop or become irregular. If spontaneous delivery of twin B is planned, be prepared to initiate oxytocin soon after the birth of the first twin (e.g., start at a rate of 3 miu/minute, doubling the rate every 5 minutes until regular contractions, maximum infusion rate of 20 miu/minute). The oxytocin should be started only after the lie of twin B has been confirmed as longitudinal. Delay amniotomy until the presenting part is longitudinal and low in the pelvis. With regular contractions, the presenting part will descend and, once fixed in the pelvis, artificial rupture of the membranes can be safely performed during a contraction. Provided the EFM is normal, allow natural progress to a vaginal delivery (either cephalic or breech).

The goal is delivery of the second twin within 30 minutes of the first. However, if there is delay and an assisted birth is required it may still be better to wait for spontaneous descent of the presenting part before performing artificial rupture of the membranes and intervening to assist the birth as long as the FHR is normal.

Several studies reviewing outcomes after external cephalic version compared with internal podalic version conclude there are no differences in neonatal or maternal outcomes. Internal podalic version followed by breech extraction is associated with a higher rate of success of vaginal birth and lower cesarean section rates.

External cephalic version

The ultrasound probe can be used as a "hand" so that fetal lie and heart rate are monitored throughout when attempting external cephalic version (Figure 12.6).

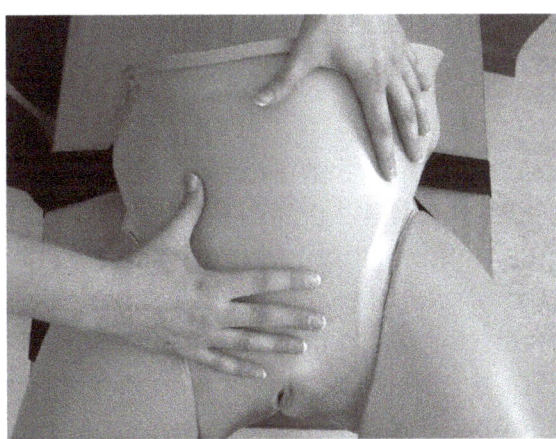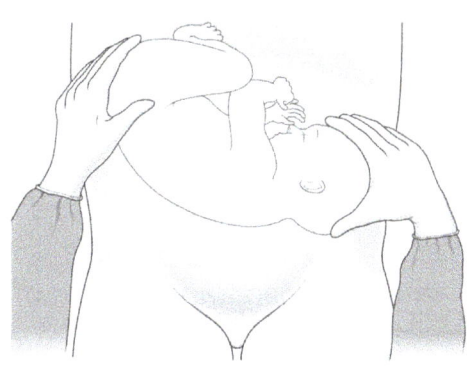

Figure 12.6 External cephalic version

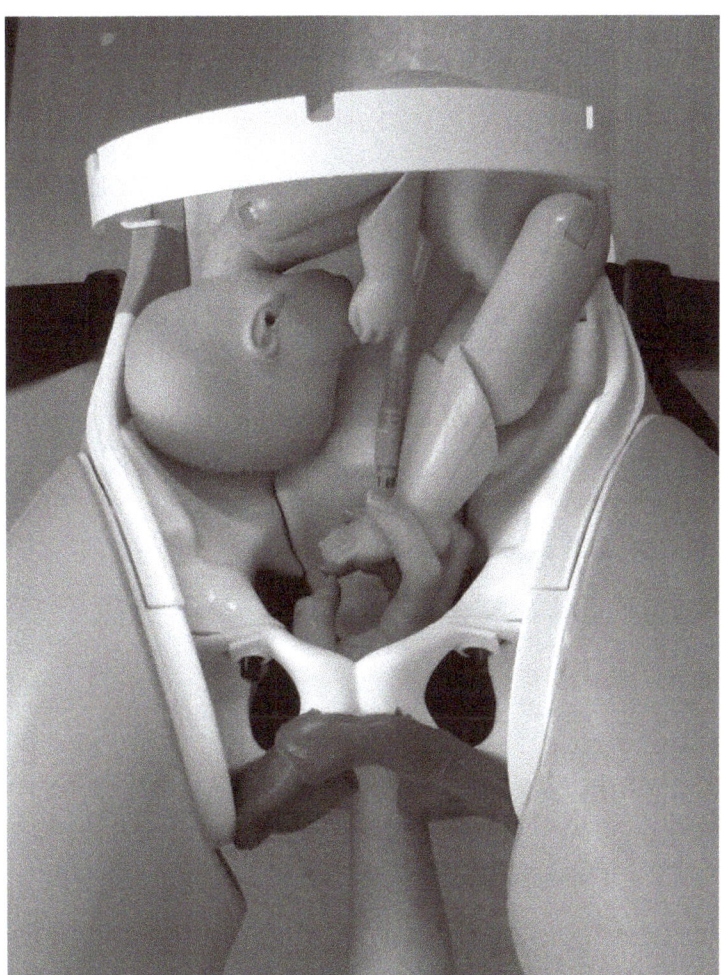

Figure 12.7 Internal podalic version

Internal podalic version

With internal podalic version, one or both fetal feet are grasped inside the uterus before proceeding to a breech extraction (Figure 12.7). Before any traction is applied, the operator must confirm that they are holding a foot by feeling the heel. It is important to try not to rupture the membranes too early, in order to avoid cord prolapse.

The same maneuvers used for an assisted breech birth may be needed to assist birth of the second twin. It is important to check the estimated fetal weights from the last growth ultrasound scan. Remember that twins are likely to be smaller than singleton fetuses. In cases of preterm twins, an incompletely dilated cervix can trap the head of a breech baby, and this risk increases as time grows after the birth of the first twin. For this reason, some practioners prefer to immediately deliver Twin B if non-cephalic in presentation. Note that the second twin may be considerably bigger (>20%) than the first twin, and this too can cause problems during birth. Under this circumstance, it is best to avoid breech extraction.

The duration of inter-twin birth interval

The duration of the inter-twin birth interval varies. Although a longer inter-twin birth interval is associated with a continuous slow decline in umbilical cord pH, the small differences in pH between 15 and 30 minutes were not large enough to alter clinical management.[9] It is generally accepted that the interval should ideally be no longer than 30 minutes.

There are theoretical concerns of acute inter-fetal transfusion in monochorionic twins following the birth of the first twin. These risks have not been substantiated; however, it remains prudent to clamp the cord of the first twin as soon as possible after its birth.[10]

Third stage of labor

Double-clamp the umbilical cord following each delivery and place an additional cord clamp on the placental end of the cord of twin B so it can be identified. Paired umbilical cord samples for blood gas measurements should be taken from the cords of both twins.

A bolus of oxytocin should be given immediately after the birth of twin B due to the high risk of postpartum hemorrhage. An oxytocin infusion should then be initiated and run according to local protocol. It is very important to continue to observe the mother for signs of postpartum hemorrhage.

As with all complicated deliveries, careful and precise documentation is paramount. Figure 12.8 is an example of a template containing the desired information.

Name:	Hospital Number:		Date:
Gestation:			Comments:
Chorionicity	Dichorionic/diamniotic or Monochorionic/diamniotic		
	Twin A	**Twin B**	
Presentation at start of 2nd stage	Vertex Breech Other	Vertex Breech Other	
EFM	Normal (I) Suspicious (II) Abnormal (III)	Normal (I) Suspicious (II) Abnormal (III)	
Oxytocin infusion	Yes No	Yes No	
Analgesia	None Narcotic Epidural Spinal GA	None Narcotic Epidural Spinal GA	
Ranitidine	Yes: Oral No	IV	
Labor nurse present	Yes Name: No		
Labor nurse present	Yes Name: No		
Obstetrician present	Yes Name: No		
Obstetrician present	Yes Name: No		
Experienced neonatologist present at birth	Yes Name: No		
Mode of birth twin A Time:	Spontaneous vaginal Vacuum Forceps LSCS		
Oxytocin infusion between twins	Yes	No	
Mode of birth twin B Time:	Spontaneous vaginal Vacuum Forceps LSCS Assisted breech Breech extraction		
	Twin A	**Twin B**	
Presentation at birth	Vertex Breech Other	Vertex Breech Other	
Internal or external maneuver performed	Yes: No	Yes: No	
Cord gases taken	Yes No	Yes No	
Apgars (at 1, 5, 10 minutes)			
Date: Name:	Signature:		

Figure 12.8 Example of a documentation template to record a twin birth

References

1. Hofmeyr GJ, Barrett JF, Crowther CA. Planned caesarean section for women with a twin pregnancy. *Cochrane Database Syst Rev* 2011; 12: CD006553.

2. Australian Institute of Health and Welfare. *Australia's Mothers and Babies 2008*. Perinatal Statistics Series No. 24. Canberra: AIHW; 2010.

3. Grisaru D, Fuchs S, Kupferminc MJ, Har-Toov J, Niv J, Lessing JB. Outcome of 306 twin deliveries according to first twin presentation and method of delivery. *Am J Perinatol* 2000; 17: 303–7.

4. Barrett JF, Hannah ME, Hutton EK, Willan AR, Allen AC, Armson BA, et al. A randomized trial of planned cesarean or vaginal delivery for twin pregnancy. *N Engl J Med* 2013; 369(14): 1295–305.

5. Hannah ME, Hannah WJ, Hewson SA, Hodnett ED, Saigal S, Willan AR. Planned caesarean section versus planned vaginal birth for breech presentation at term: a randomised multicentre trial. Term Breech Trial Collaborative Group. *Lancet* 2000; 356: 1375–83.

6. Tessen JA, Zlatnik FJ. Monoamniotic twins: a retrospective controlled study. *Obstet Gynecol* 1991; 77: 832–4.

7. Hartley RS, Emanuel I, Hitti J. Perinatal mortality and neonatal morbidity rates among twin pairs at different gestational ages: optimal delivery timing at 37 to 38 weeks' gestation. *Am J Obstet Gynecol* 2001; 184: 451–8.

8. Royal College of Obstetricians and Gynaecologists. *Management of Monochorionic Twin Pregnancy*. Green-top Guideline No. 51. London: RCOG; 2008 [www.rcog.org.uk/womens-health/clinical-guidance/management-monochorionic-twin-pregnancy].

9. McGrail CD, Bryant DR. Intertwin time interval: how it affects the immediate neonatal outcome of the second twin. *Am J Obstet Gynecol* 2005; 192: 1420–2.

10. Wright CE, Chauhan SP, Abuhamad AZ. Bakri balloon in the management of postpartum hemorrhage: a review. *Am J Perinatol* 2014;31: 957–64.

Module 13
Acute uterine inversion

Key learning points

- Recognize an inverted uterus and the accompanying maternal shock.
- Call for appropriate help and immediately manage the maternal shock.
- Be able to outline the mechanical maneuvers to replace the uterus, including manually replacing the uterus as soon as possible.
- Emphasize the placenta should not be removed, if adherent, until the uterus has been replaced.

Common difficulties observed in training drills

- Delay recognizing the problem.
- Not stating the problem clearly to those first responding to the emergency call.
- Delay initiating resuscitation.
- Delay manually replacing the uterus.
- Not being prepared for a subsequent postpartum hemorrhage.

Introduction

Acute inversion of the uterus is a rare complication of childbirth. The incidence varies widely from 1/1,500 to 1/20,000 births.[1,2] There are no randomized controlled trials addressing the best management options, although several case reports recommend immediate replacement of the uterus as the most successful management strategy.[2]

Definition

When the uterus inverts, the fundus of the uterus descends abnormally through the genital tract, turning itself inside out. There are three grades of uterine inversion:

- Grade I: fundus inverts down to the cervical canal
- Grade II: fundus inverts into the vagina
- Grade III: fundus is visible at the introitus.

The recognized risk factors for acute uterine inversion are described in Box 13.1.[3,4]

Diagnosis

Uterine inversion can be difficult to diagnose, particularly if the fundus is not outside the introitus. The sudden development of maternal shock is often the first sign of a uterine inversion, and is frequently unexpected as there may be minimal blood loss.

Box 13.1 Risk factors for uterine inversion

Excessive traction on the umbilical cord

Inappropriate fundal pressure

Short umbilical cord

Multiparity

Abnormally adherent placenta

Vaginal birth after cesarean (VBAC)

Abnormalities of the uterus (e.g., unicornuate uterus)

Prior uterine inversion

Fetal macrosomia

Precipitate labor

Connective tissue disorders (e.g., Marfan syndrome, Ehlers–Danlos syndrome)

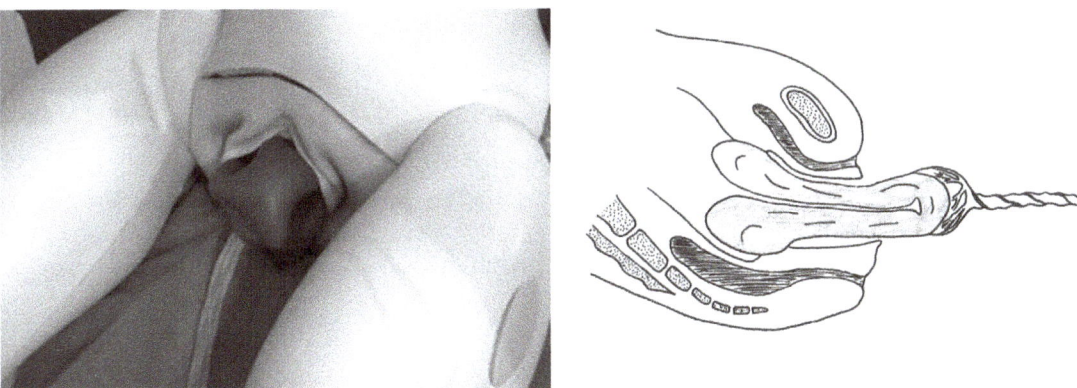

Figure 13.1 A Grade III uterine inversion

An abdominal and vaginal examination should be performed rapidly. Grade III uterine inversion is characterized by a mass (uterus) protruding through the introitus (Figure 13.1). *However, there should be a high index of suspicion for uterine inversion whenever the fundus is not palpable on abdominal exam.* As the uterus inverts through the cervix, it stimulates the vagus nerve, leading to vasovagal (neurogenic) shock, characterized by bradycardia[3] and hypotension.[4] The woman often looks as if she has fainted, but there is minimal blood loss. Hypovolemic shock with tachycardia and hypotension may also occur if postpartum hemorrhage follows the uterine inversion. *While all women should be treated with standard initial resuscitation, the quickest way to resolve neurogenic shock is to return the uterus to its anatomical position.*[3]

> **Uterine inversion is associated with atony and postpartum hemorrhage in over 90% of cases.[3,5] This occurs after the uterus has been replaced and the placenta removed. Measure the blood loss accurately to avoid an underestimation.[6]**

Management

Immediate action

Figure 13.2 offers an algorithm for the immediate management of an inverted uterus. Maternal shock should be treated immediately and appropriate help called.

- Call for help: this should include a senior obstetrical nurse, the most experienced obstetrician available, and an anesthesiologist.
- Give high-flow oxygen (10 l/minute) via a facemask with reservoir.

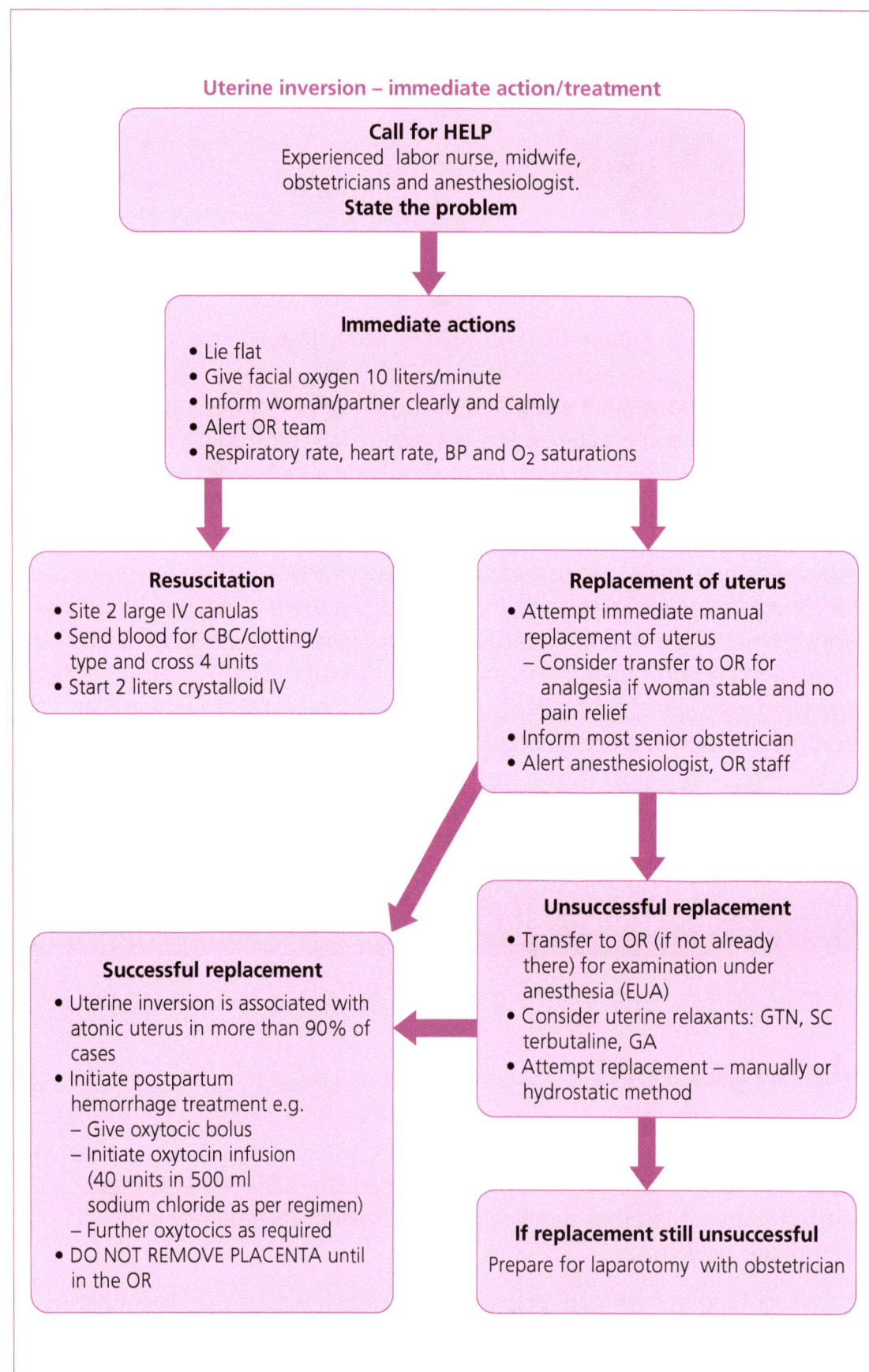

Figure 13.2 Management algorithm for acute uterine inversion

- Clearly and calmly inform the woman of the need to immediately reposition the uterine fundus.
- Treatment of uterine inversion and resuscitation should take place simultaneously.

Resuscitation

- Place two large-bore intravenous cannulas.
- Infuse 2 liters of Ringer's solution.
- Obtain blood samples for a type and cross (4 units), CBC, and a clotting profile. (The main complication of uterine inversion is atonic postpartum hemorrhage.[7])
- The quickest way to treat neurogenic shock is to replace the uterus.

Treatment

- The uterus should be replaced as soon as possible.
- If the woman is bleeding heavily, is hemodynamically unstable, or already has effective analgesia, the accoucheur should manually replace the uterus immediately in the labor room or at home.
- If the woman is stable and does not have adequate analgesia, prompt transfer to the OR for analgesia should be considered prior to replacement.
- If replacement is successful, administer an intramuscular oxytocic agent such as Hemabate or methylergonovine followed by an infusion of oxytocin 40 units in 500 ml normal saline over 4 hours.
- If uterine replacement is unsuccessful, transfer the patient to the OR.
- If a uterine inversion occurs outside the hospital:
  - ☐ Immediately attempt replacement and call an ambulance.
  - ☐ If the uterus is successfully replaced, an oxytoxic should be administered and the woman still transferred to the hospital.
  - ☐ If the uterus is not replaced, the woman should be transferred to the nearest obstetric unit as quickly as possible. The hospital should be informed so that the OR team is ready on the woman's arrival.

Management of the inversion

The uterus can be manually replaced by putting a hand into the vagina and following the cord to the fundus; while supporting the inverted fundus in the palm of the hand, gently raise the uterus into the abdominal cavity and

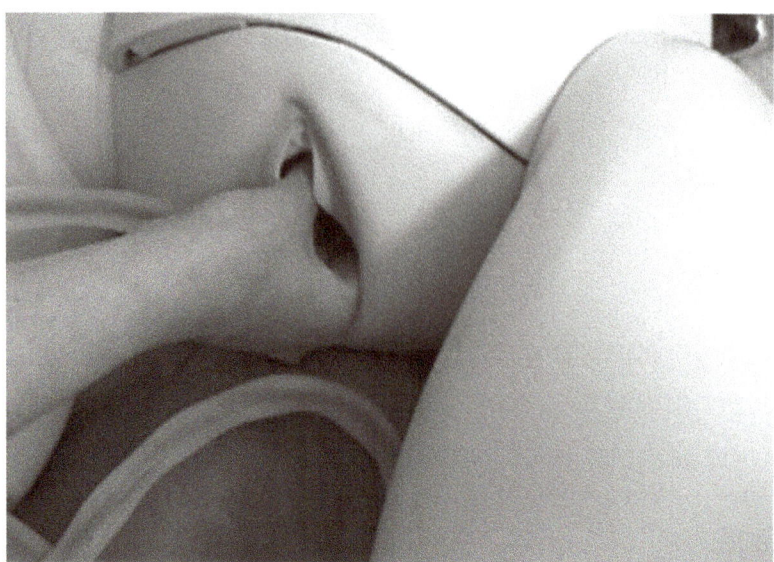

Figure 13.3 Manual replacement of the inverted uterus

"replace" it back to its anatomical position (Figure 13.3). If the placenta is still attached, do not remove it before uterine replacement.[2]

The earlier the replacement is attempted, the more likely it is to be successful.[5] The uterus becomes edematous as it remains prolapsed, and a constriction ring may develop making replacement more difficult.[3]

Uterine relaxants

Tocolysis can be useful to relax the uterus to assist manual replacement particularly if a constriction ring has developed. Terbutaline (250 mcg subcutaneously) or glyceryl trinitrate spray (one metered dose sublingually) may be used for this purpose. General anesthesia may also promote uterine relaxation and can be useful if repeat attempts at uterine replacement are necessary.

> **Caution should be exercised with the use of uterine relaxants as they will exacerbate atonic postpartum hemorrhage once the uterus is replaced.**

Hydrostatic method for the management of an inverted uterus

As an alternative to surgery, uterine inversion may be corrected using hydrostatic pressure to distend the vagina and push the fundus upward into its anatomical position. This technique was originally described by simply sealing the vaginal entrance with an assistant's hand;[8] however, a silastic

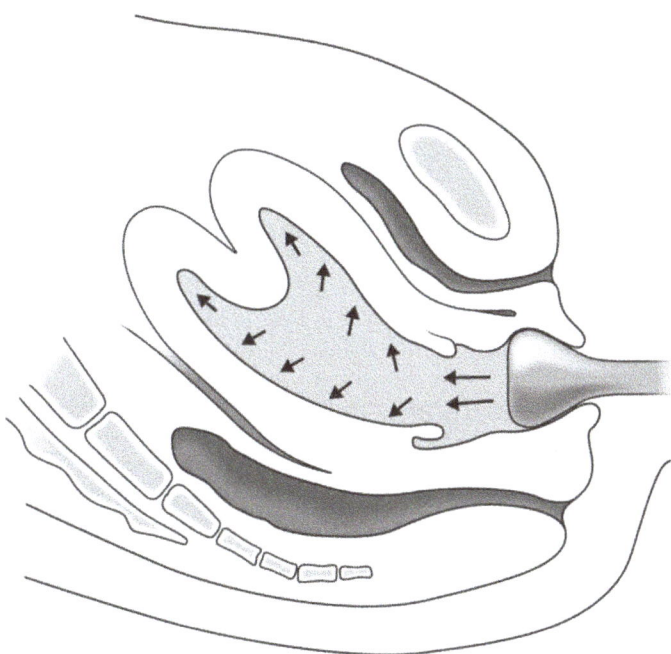

Figure 13.4 Hydrostatic method for the management of an inverted uterus

vacuum cup can be used to create a better seal, thus improving the hydrostatic pressure (Figure 13.4).[9]

Equipment required:

- vacuum cup
- blood-administration set
- 2 liters of warm normal saline intravenous solution.

The vacuum cup is placed into the vagina so as to occlude the vaginal opening. Two liters of body temperature intravenous normal saline are rapidly infused using the blood administration set, which is attached directly to the end of the vacuum cup. The fluid bag held 10 to 15 inches above the level of the vagina to provide sufficient pressure for insufflation. Reduction of the inversion is usually achieved within 5 to 10 minutes.

Continuing management

Once the uterus is successfully replaced, it should be manually held in position for a few minutes to promote uterine contraction and prevent re-inversion.[3] The use of a Bakri tamponade balloon catheter (Cook® Medical Incorporated, Bloomington, IN, USA) has also used after replacement of the uterus for the same purpose, with the added benefit of treating atony.[10] Oxytocics should be administered at this point, with an initial bolus dose and an infusion over 4 hours.

If the placenta is adherent, it should be manually removed after the uterus has been replaced.

Broad-spectrum antibiotics are given with manual uterine replacement and continued for 24 hours, in line with local practices.

Surgical management

Laparotomy may be required in rare circumstances when the above techniques are unsuccessful. Upward traction on the uterus using the round ligaments is used to achieve replacement to the anatomical position. If this procedure is unsuccessful, one can vertically incise the ring of cervical edema posteriorly to aid replacement of the uterus.[3]

Documentation

It is important that all personnel involved and treatments administered are documented in the medical record as soon after the event as possible.

Debriefing after the emergency

Once the patient's clinical condition is stable and she is comfortable, she needs to be debriefed about the sudden event. This is best undertaken by one of the members of the team that managed the clinical problem. The woman may need to be told that:

■ it is difficult to predict recurrence, as experience with uterine inversion is limited

■ hospital birth and active management of the 3rd stage of labor is recommended for future pregnancies

■ uterine inversion can occur outside pregnancy and childbirth.

References

1. Hussain M, Jabeen T, Liaquat N, Noorani K, Bhutta SZ. Acute puerperal uterine inversion. *J Coll Physicians Surg Pak* 2004; 14: 215–17.

2. Milenkovic M, Kahn J. Inversion of the uterus: a serious complication at childbirth. *Acta Obstet Gynecol Scand* 2005; 84: 95–6.

3. Bhalla R, Wuntakal R, Odejinmi F, Khan RU. Acute inversion of the uterus. *The Obstetrician & Gynaecologist* 2009; 11: 13–18.

4. Belfort M, Dildy G. Postpartum haemorrhage and other problems of the third stage. In James DK, Steer PJ, Weiner CP, Gonik B (eds) *High Risk Pregnancy: Management Options, 4th edn.* London: Saunders; 2011.

5. Watson P, Besch N, Bowes WA Jr. Management of acute and subacute puerperal inversion of the uterus. *Obstet Gynecol* 1980; 55: 12–16.

6. Beringer RM, Patteril M. Puerperal uterine inversion and shock. *Br J Anaesth* 2004; 92: 439–41.

7. Baskett TF. Acute uterine inversion: a review of 40 cases. *J Obstet Gynaecol Can* 2002; 24: 953–6.

8. O'Sullivan JV. Acute inversion of the uterus.*Br Med J* 1945; 2: 282–3.

9. Ogueh O, Ayida G. Acute uterine inversion: a new technique of hydrostatic replacement. *BJOG* 1997; 104: 951–2.

10. Soleymani Majd S, Pilsniak A, Reginald PW. Recurrent uterine inversion: a novel treatment approach using SOS Bakri balloon. *BJOG* 2009; 116: 999–1001.

Module 14
Basic newborn resuscitation

Key learning points

- Develop and practice a structured approach to the skills required for neonatal resuscitation.

- Understand the causes of respiratory and cardiac arrest in the neonate and anticipate problems attributable to maternal obstetric history.

- Understand the importance of calling for help early.

- Communicate effectively with the parents and the neonatal team.

- Complete and accurate documentation.

Difficulties observed in previous neonatal resuscitation drills

- Lack of attention to temperature during resuscitation, especially in preterm infants.

- Failure to open the infant's airway adequately, usually due to over-extension of the neck.

- Loss of an effective airway, particularly when conducting simultaneous cardiac compressions.

- Performing chest compressions too slowly.

Introduction

This module provides an outline of the process of basic newborn resuscitation but is not intended to be a complete guide. Further information is available from the Neonatal Resuscitation Program sponsored jointly by the American Heart Association and the American Academy of Pediatrics.[1]

Background

All neonates experience a degree of hypoxia during labor and delivery, with respiratory exchange being interrupted for as long as 50 to 75 seconds with each contraction during labor. The norm is a lactate acidosis compared to the prelabor baseline. And while most healthy babies tolerate it well, some do not and require additional help to establish normal breathing once born.[1,2]

The fetus is designed to tolerate the stress of labor, and the neonate's brain can withstand much longer periods without oxygen than an adult brain. In addition, the neonatal heart can continue to beat effectively for 20 minutes or more without lung aeration, even after the reserve system of gasping has ceased. Therefore the primary aim of newborn resuscitation is to inflate the lungs with air or oxygen so the still functioning circulation can deliver oxygenated blood to and from the heart.[1, 2]

Physiology of neonatal hypoxia

There are two centers in the brain that control respiration; one is a higher center. If the hypoxic insult to the fetus is severe, *in utero* breathing movements become deeper, more rapid, but eventually cease, as the centers responsible for controlling them are unable to function due to the lack of oxygen. This is known as "primary apnea."[1,2]

Once the baby develops "primary apnea," the heart rate falls to about half its usual rate as the heart muscle switches from aerobic to the less efficient anaerobic metabolism. Lactic acid derived from anaerobic metabolism now builds rapidly causing the newborn baby to become acidotic and the circulation is diverted away from non-essential organs. After a variable length of time of continuing hypoxia, unconscious gasping activity is initiated. The baby begins shuddering, a whole-body gasp at about 12 breaths/minute.[3] If these gasps fail to aerate the lungs, breathing ceases altogether, leading to "secondary" or "terminal apnea." At this point, the baby becomes increasingly acidotic and the heart begins to fail. If there is no effective intervention, the baby will die (*in utero* if unborn or *ex utero* if already born) and may even die despite treatment.[1] The whole process takes about 20 minutes in a newborn baby.[4]

While the heart continues to beat, the most important part of neonatal resuscitation is aerating the lungs so that oxygenated blood can be delivered to the heart and, hence, the brain and the respiratory centers. Unfortunately, it is not possible to tell at birth whether a newborn who is not breathing is in primary apnea and about to gasp, or is in the terminal apnea phase. In most cases, the infant will quickly recover once air enters the lungs and normal breathing will begin. A few babies may require cardiac massage, but usually for only a short period of time.[1]

A few babies born at the point of terminal apnea will die without intervention, and may die despite it. In addition to ventilation and cardiac massage, drugs may be required to restore the circulation. By this stage, an experienced neonatologist should be in attendance and lead the resuscitation. If drugs are required, the general outlook is poor.

Preparation of resuscitation equipment

Successful resuscitation is dependent on forward planning. Before any birth, it is the responsibility of the nurse and/or the neonatologist responsible for resuscitation to prepare and check resuscitation equipment:

- clock and light
- air and suction (cylinders full and suction tubing attached)
- neonatal warmer and prewarmed towels and hat
- equipment for administering air (bag/valve mask and appropriately sized mask, T-piece tubing)
- neonatal laryngoscopes (correct size blades and light working)
- notes for documentation.

Consider the woman's obstetric history when preparing for a delivery, and call the neonatal team in advance, if indicated. It is important to explain to the parents that a neonatologist has been called and to keep them informed of the situation.

Delayed cord clamping

The Neonatal Resuscitation Program (NRP) guideline recommends delayed cord clamping for at least 1 minute after the delivery of an uncompromised infant.[1] For healthy term infants, delaying cord clamping for at least 1 minute or until the cord stops pulsating improves iron status through early infancy.[1] The level at which the baby should be held in relation to the mother when delaying cord clamping in order to achieve the optimal speed and amount of placental blood transfusion is unspecified. In one study, the baby was held about 20 cm below the mother for approximately 30 seconds before placing the baby on the mother's abdomen.[5]

Taking into consideration the risk of hypothermia in the wet newborn, the infant should be dried, kept warm, and assessed for color, tone, breathing, and heart rate while waiting to clamp the cord. There is insufficient evidence to recommend an appropriate time for clamping the cord in newborns that are severely compromised at birth. Therefore resuscitative interventions remain a priority.

Assessment and resuscitation

As in any emergency, it is important to call for help early. An outline of basic newborn resuscitation is shown in Figure 14.1, but this is not intended to be a complete guide. Further information is available from the NPR Manual or STABLE.[1,2]

1. Warmth and assessment at birth

Newborn babies have a large surface area to body ratio and are wet at birth. They rapidly lose heat and, if hypoxic and/or small, can quickly become hypothermic.[6]

At delivery:

- Start the clock and note the time of birth.
- Dry the baby, remove any wet towels, and then wrap in warm dry towels; place a hat on. Drying the baby both stimulates neonatal respirations and provides time for a full assessment of color, tone, respiratory effort, and heart rate (Figures 14.2 and 14.3).
- For uncompromised babies, delay cord clamping for at least 1 minute from the complete birth of the infant. After 1 minute, the cord should be securely clamped.

> **Resuscitative intervention remains the priority in babies who require resuscitation – do not delay cord clamping if this will interfere with neonatal resuscitation.**

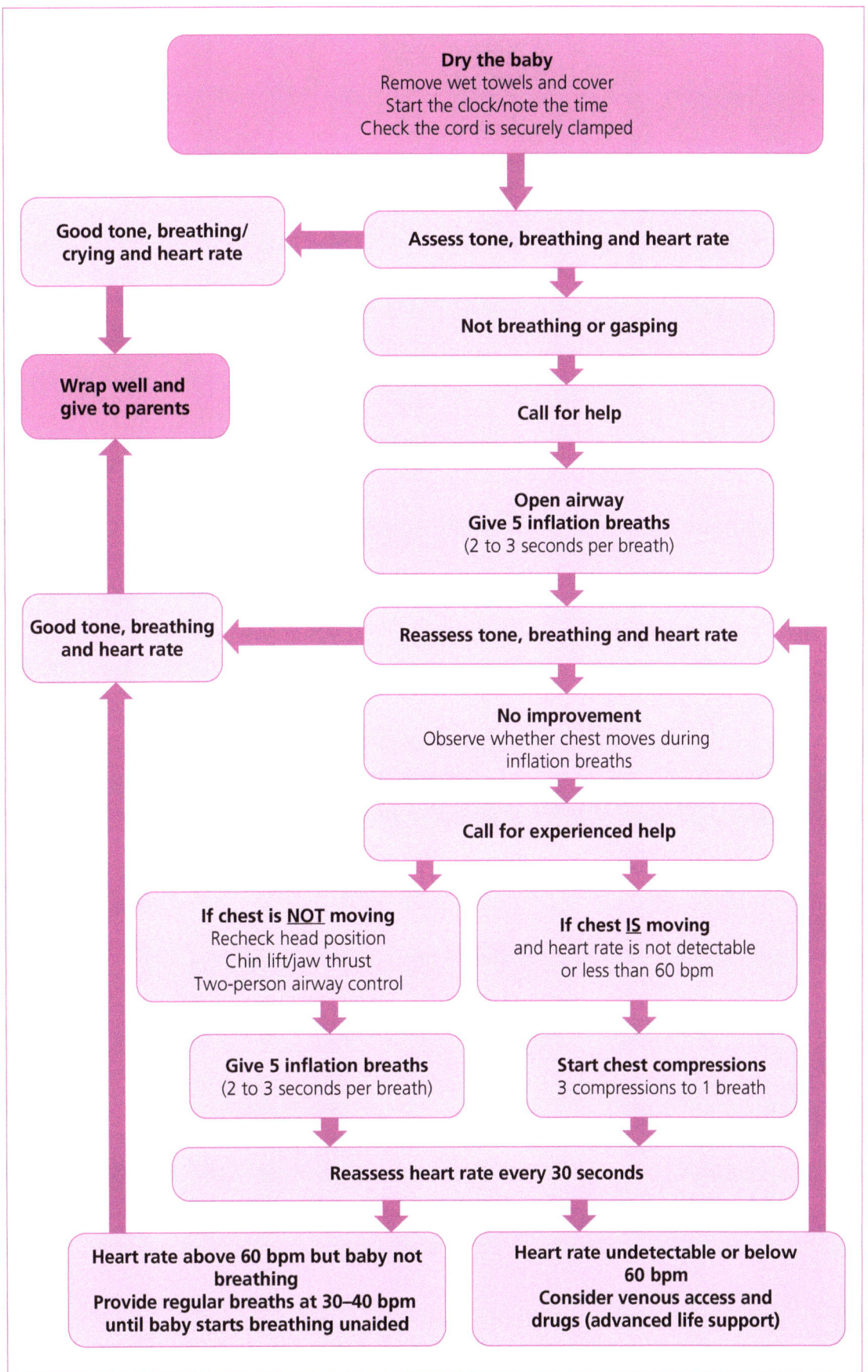

Figure 14.1 Modified newborn life support algorithm

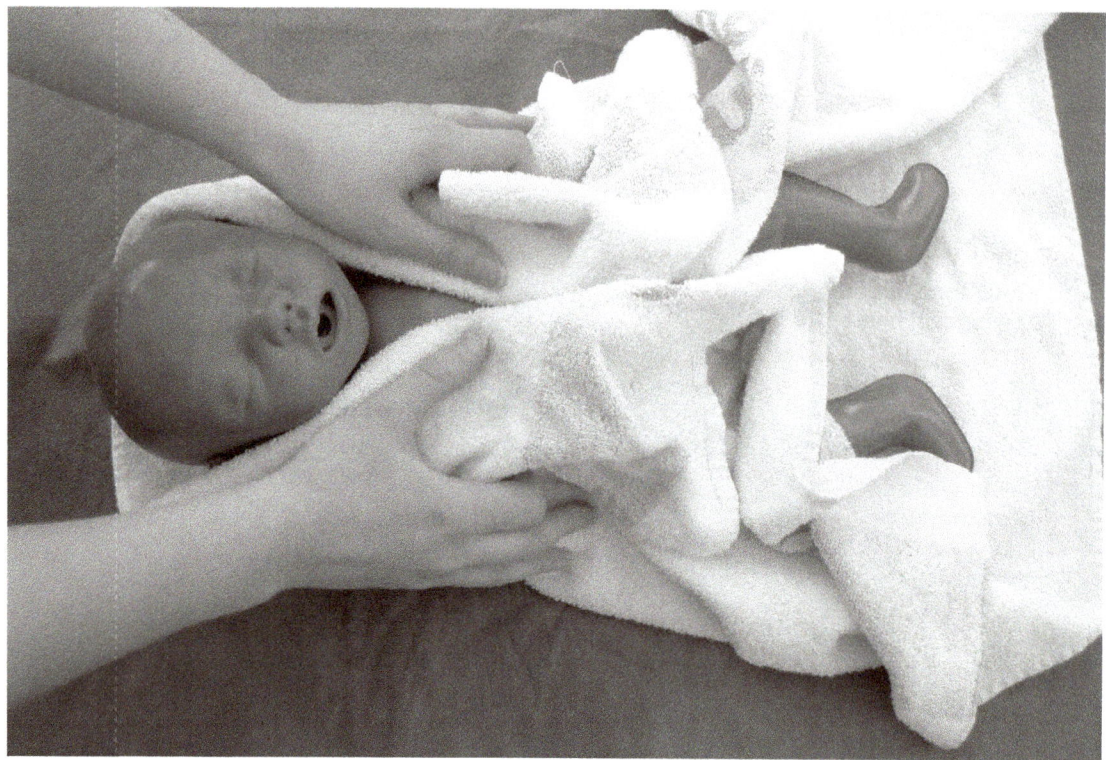

Figure 14.2 Dry the baby with a warm towel

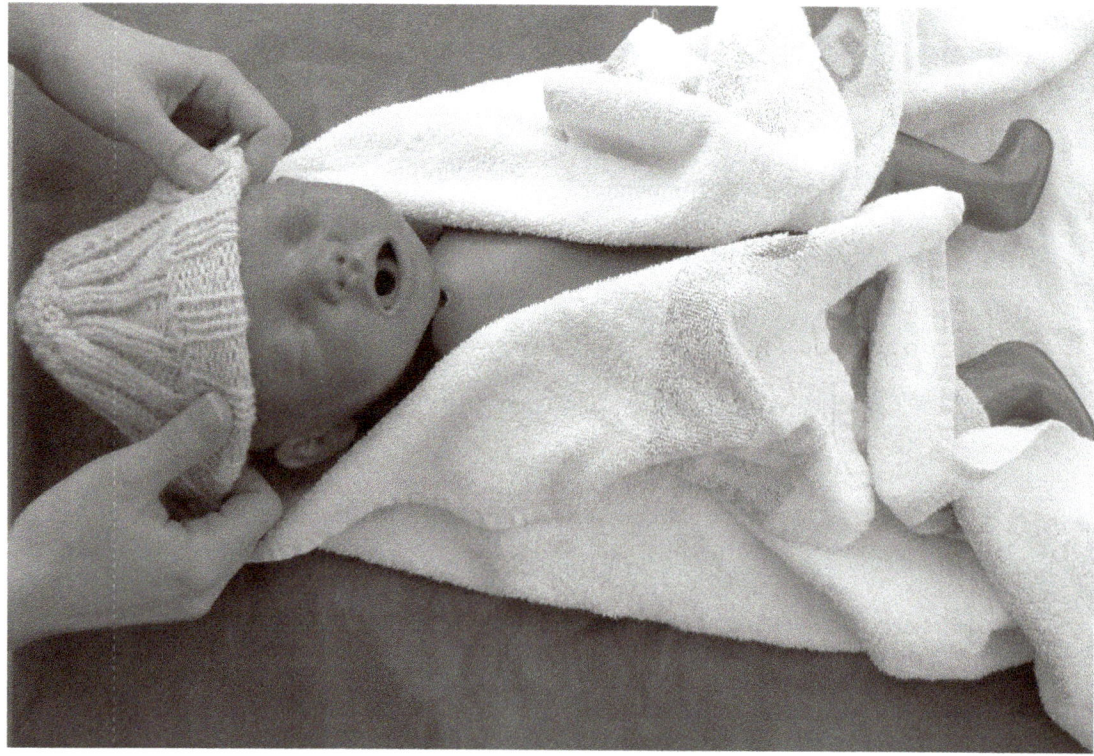

Figure 14.3 Wrap the baby in a warm dry towel and put a hat on the baby

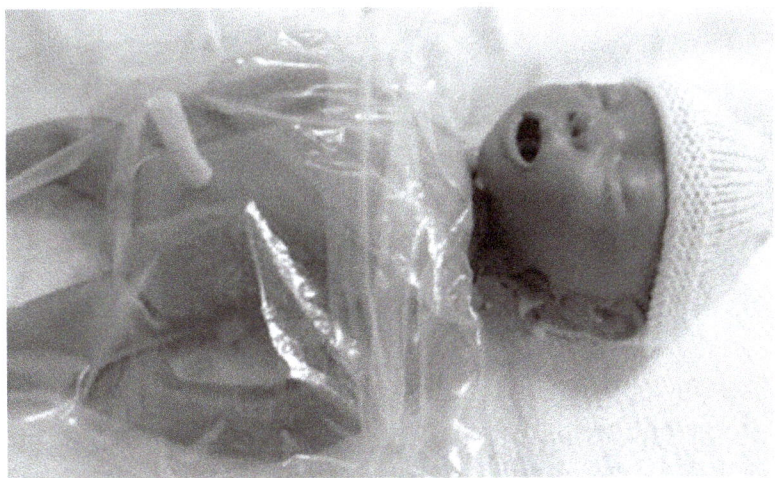

Figure 14.4 Preterm baby placed in a food bag

- A healthy baby will be born blue but with good tone, cry, and have a good heart rate all within a few seconds of birth (the heart rate of a healthy newborn baby is about 120 to 150 bpm).

- A less healthy baby will be blue at birth, have low tone, may have a slow heart rate (below than 100 bpm) and not establish adequate breathing by 90 to 120 seconds.

- An ill baby will be born pale and floppy, not breathing, and have a slow, very slow, or undetectable heart rate.

Preterm babies born at less than 28 weeks should not be dried at birth, but rather immediately covered up to their necks in a food-grade plastic wrap or bag (Figure 14.4). The labor room temperature should be at least 26°C and the neonate placed under a radiant heater and stabilized. This is a very effective method of keeping preterm infants warm. They should remain wrapped until their temperature has been checked after admission to the NICU.

2. Airway

Most newborns have a prominent occiput, which causes them to flex their neck if placed flat on their backs; this in turn blocks their airway (Figure 14.5). To avoid this, babies should be placed on their back with their head in a neutral position (Figure 14.6). It may help to place some support under the shoulders to maintain this position.

If the baby is very floppy, a chin lift or jaw thrust may also be necessary to keep the airway open (Figure 14.7).

Airway suction immediately following delivery is seldom necessary and should be reserved for babies with obvious airway obstruction that cannot be

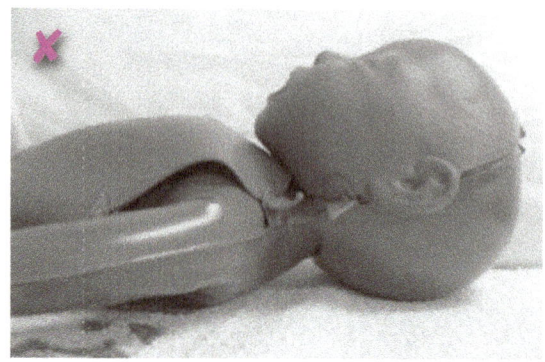

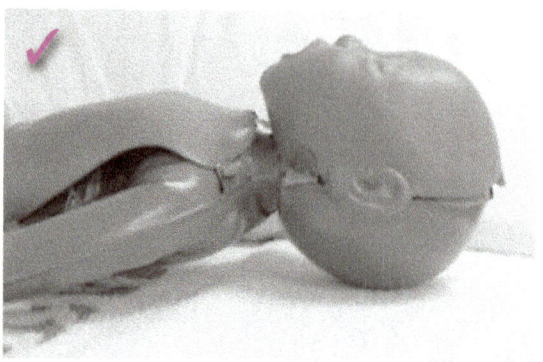

Figure 14.5 Airway obstruction caused by prominent occiput

Figure 14.6 Head in the neutral position, opening the airway

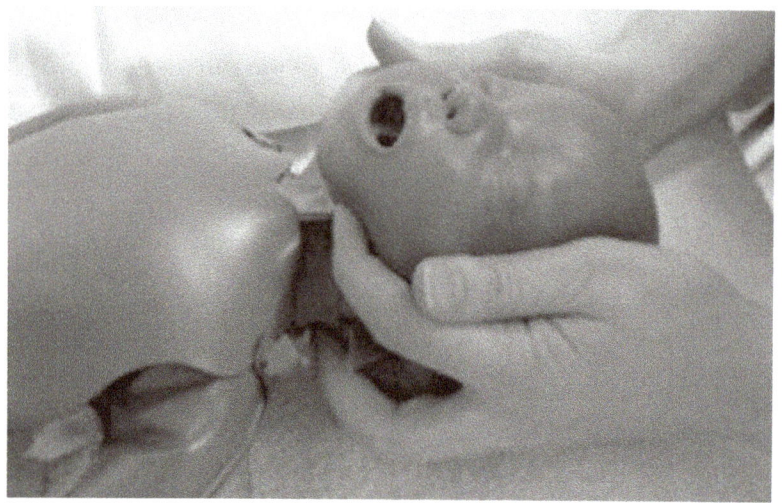

Figure 14.7 Chin lift and jaw thrust to open the airway

overcome by the appropriate head positioning noted above. Rarely, material may block the oropharynx or trachea. In these situations, direct visualization and suction of the oropharynx should be performed. For tracheal obstruction, intubation and suction on withdrawal of the endotracheal tube may be effective but should be attempted only by an experienced practitioner.

3. Breathing

If the newborn is not breathing adequately within about 90 seconds, five inflatory breaths (of air) should be given. It is important the correct mask size be used: covering the chin, but not over the eyes or squeezing the nose (Figure 14.8). The baby's lungs are filled with fluid at birth, so the inflation breaths will force out the fluid and fill the lungs with air. The pressure required to initially inflate the lungs is equivalent to 30 cm of water for 2 to 3 seconds/breath.[1]

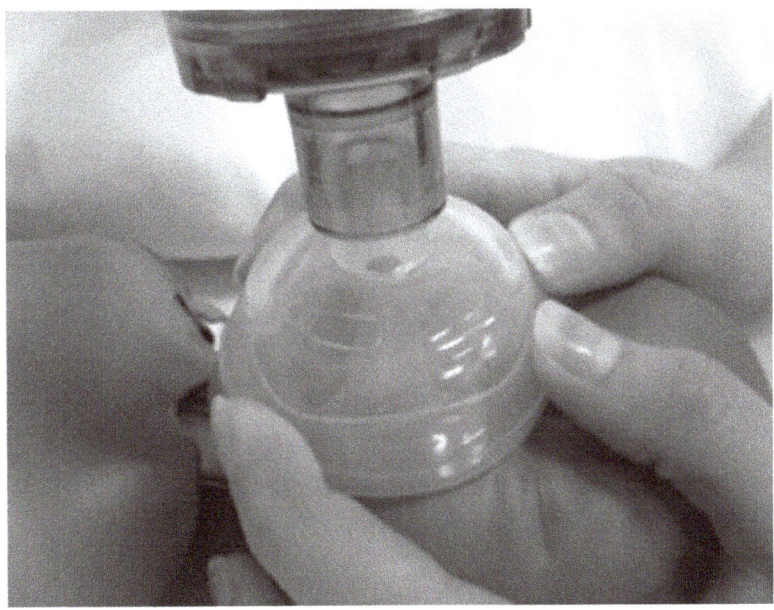

Figure 14.8 Inflation breaths using correct-sized facemask covering the nose and mouth

If the lungs have been effectively inflated, passive movements of the chest wall will be visible and the heart rate should also increase as oxygenated blood reaches the heart. If the heart rate increases but the baby does not start breathing on his/her own, regular ventilation breaths at a rate of 30 to 40/minute should be continued until the baby begins to breathe spontaneously.

If the heart rate does not increase following inflation breaths, it may be because the baby needs more than lung aeration. But a more likely explanation is that the lungs were not effectively aerated. Therefore go back to the beginning, check the airway, make sure the baby's head is in the neutral position with a jaw thrust if necessary, and confirm there is no obstruction in the oropharynx. If the chest wall still does not move, request assistance in maintaining the airway and consider intubating the newborn.

If the heart rate remains slow or is absent despite five good inflation breaths with passive chest movement, chest compressions are needed and neonatal support should be requested.

4. Chest compression/circulation

Almost all babies needing resuscitation at birth respond successfully to lung inflation, with a rise in heart rate proceeding rapidly to normal breathing. However, in some cases chest compression is necessary. It is important that chest compression be initiated only when it is certain the lungs have been

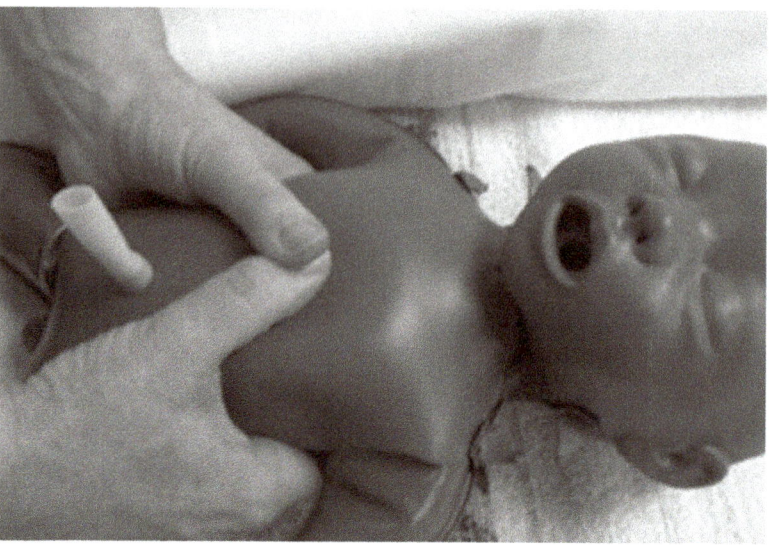

Figure 14.9 Positioning for chest compressions

successfully inflated. Neonatal support should be urgently summoned if not already in attendance.

The most efficient way to perform chest compressions in an infant is to grip the chest with both hands, with both thumbs pressing on the lower third of the sternum, just below the nipple line, and the fingers over the spine at the back (Figure 14.9).

Compress the chest quickly and firmly to a depth of about one-third of the distance from the chest to the spine. The ratio of compressions to breaths recommended in a newborn infant is 3:1 to achieve 90 compressions and 30 breaths in one minute. Allow enough time between compressions for oxygenated blood to flow from the lungs to the heart at a rate of approximately 120 events/minute. Be sure that the chest is inflating with each ventilatory breath. In a very small number of babies, lung inflation and chest compressions will not be sufficient to generate an effective circulation and, in such circumstances, drugs may be required.

5. Meconium at delivery

There is no evidence that suctioning meconium from the nose and mouth of the infant while the head is still on the perineum prevents meconium aspiration; this outmoded practice is not recommended.[7] In addition, attempting to remove meconium from the airways of a vigorously crying infant has also been proved to be ineffective at preventing meconium aspiration.[8] However, if a baby is born unresponsive and there is thick meconium present, the oropharynx should be suctioned to clear the meconium. If an individual skilled in intubation is available, the larynx and trachea should also be cleared. However, if the attempted intubation is prolonged or unsuccessful, it is important to start mask ventilation, particularly if there is persistent bradycardia.

6. Emergency drugs

Emergency drugs are needed only if there is no significant circulatory response despite effective ventilation and chest compressions. An experienced neonatologist should be in attendance at this stage and it is their responsibility to intubate the infant and administer medication.

7. Therapeutic hypothermia

In a newborn that is at or near term, where moderate or severe hypoxic ischemic encephalopathy (HIE) is a possibility, an experienced neonatologist may consider treatment with therapeutic hypothermia. If this is the case, the heater of the infant warmer should be switched off.[1]

Documentation

It is important that all actions are documented accurately and comprehensively in the medical record, particularly when resuscitation at birth has been necessary, as records may be carefully scrutinized many years later.

References

1. *Neonatal Resuscitation, 5th edn.* American Academy of Pediatrics and the American Heart Association; 2011.
2. Karlsen, K. *STABLE, 6th edn.* Kristen A Karlsen; 2013.
3. Dawes G. *Fetal and Neonatal Physiology.* Chicago: Year Book Publisher; 1968, pp. 141–59.
4. Hey E, Kelly J. Gaseous exchange during endotracheal ventilation for asphyxia at birth. *J Obstet Gynaecol Br Commonw* 1968; 75: 414–23.
5. Andersson O, Hellström-Westas L, Andersson D, Domellöf M. Effect of delayed versus early umbilical cord clamping on neonatal outcomes and iron status at 4 months: a randomised controlled trial. *BMJ* 2011; 343: d7157.
6. Dahm LS, James LS. Newborn temperature and calculated heat loss in the delivery room. *Pediatrics* 1972; 49: 504–13.
7. Vain NE, Szyld EG, Prudent LM, Wiswell TE, Aguilar AM, Vivas NI. Oropharyngeal and nasopharyngeal suctioning of meconium-stained neonates before delivery of their shoulders: multicentre, randomised controlled trial. *Lancet* 2004; 364: 597–602.
8. Wiswell TE, Gannon CM, Jacob J, Goldsmith L, Szyld E, Weiss K, et al. Delivery room management of the apparently vigorous meconium-stained neonate: results of the multicenter, international collaborative trial. *Pediatrics* 2000; 105: 1–7.

Index

For EU product safety concerns, contact us at Calle de José Abascal, 56–1°,
28003 Madrid, Spain or eugpsr@cambridge.org.

www.ingramcontent.com/pod-product-compliance
Ingram Content Group UK Ltd.
Pitfield, Milton Keynes, MK11 3LW, UK
UKHW050452090126
466816UK00016B/274